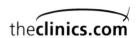

MEDICAL CLINICS
OF NORTH AMERICA

Pain Management, Part I

GUEST EDITOR
Howard S. Smith, MD

January 2007 • Volume 91 • Number 1

SAUNDERS

An Imprint of Elsevier, Inc.
PHILADELPHIA LONDON TORONTO MONTREAL SYDNEY TOKYO

W.B. SAUNDERS COMPANY
A Division of Elsevier Inc.

1600 John F. Kennedy Boulevard • Suite 1800 • Philadelphia, Pennsylvania 19103-2899

http://www.theclinics.com

MEDICAL CLINICS OF NORTH AMERICA Volume 91, Number 1
January 2007 ISSN 0025-7125
Editor: Rachel Glover ISBN-13: 978-1-4160-4334-8
  ISBN-10: 1-4160-4334-9

Medical Clinics of North America (ISSN 0025-7125) is published bimonthly by W.B. Saunders, 360 Park Avenue South, New York, NY 10010-1710. Business and editorial offices: 1600 John F. Kennedy Boulevard, Suite 1800, Philadelphia, PA 19103-2899. Accounting and circulation offices: 6277 Sea Harbor Drive, Orlando, FL 32887-4800. Periodicals postage paid at New York, NY, and additional mailing offices. Subscription prices are USD 157 per year for US individuals, USD 273 per year for US institutions, USD 81 per year for US students, USD 200 per year for Canadian individuals, USD 347 per year for Canadian institutions, USD 119 per year for Canadian students, USD 227 per year for international individuals, USD 347 per year for international institutions and USD 119 per year for international students. To receive student/resident rate, orders must be accompanied by name of affiliated institution, date of term, and the *signature* of program/residency coordinator on institution letterhead. Orders will be billed at individual rate until proof of status is received. Foreign air speed delivery is included in all *Clinics* subscription prices. All prices are subject to change without notice. POSTMASTER: Send address changes to *Medical Clinics of North America*, Elsevier Periodicals Customer Service, 6277 Sea Harbor Drive, Orlando, FL 32887-4800. **Customer Service: 1-800-654-2452 (US). From outside of the USA, call (+1) 407-345-1000. E-mail: hhspcs@harcourt.com.**

Reprints. For copies of 100 or more, of articles in this publication, please contact the Commercial Reprints Department, Elsevier Inc., 360 Park Avenue South, New York, New York 10010-1710. Tel.: (+1) 212) 633-3813; Fax: (+1) (212) 462-1935; E-mail: reprints@elsevier.com.

Medical Clinics of North America is also published in Spanish by McGraw-Hill Interamericana Editores S. A., P.O. Box 5-237, 06500 Mexico, D.F., Mexico.

Medical Clinics of North America is covered in *Index Medicus, Current Contents, ASCA, Excerpta Medica, Science Citation Index,* and *ISI/BIOMED.*

Printed in the United States of America.

GOAL STATEMENT

The goal of *Medical Clinics of North America* is to keep practicing physicians up to date with current clinical practice by providing timely articles reviewing the state of the art in patient care.

ACCREDITATION

The *Medical Clinics of North America* is planned and implemented in accordance with the Essential Areas and Policies of the Accreditation Council for Continuing Medical Education (ACCME) through the joint sponsorship of the University of Virginia School of Medicine and Elsevier. The University of Virginia School of Medicine is accredited by the ACCME to provide continuing medical education for physicians.

The University of Virginia School of Medicine designates this educational activity for a maximum of 90 *AMA PRA Category 1 Credits™*. Physicians should only claim credit commensurate with the extent of their participation in the activity.

The American Medical Association has determined that physicians not licensed in the US who participate in this CME activity are eligible for *AMA PRA Category 1 Credits™*.

Credit can be earned by reading the text material, taking the CME examination online at http://www.theclinics.com/home/cme, and completing the evaluation. After taking the test, you will be required to review any and all incorrect answers. Following completion of the test and evaluation, your credit will be awarded and you may print your certificate.

FACULTY DISCLOSURE/CONFLICT OF INTEREST

The University of Virginia School of Medicine, as an ACCME accredited provider, endorses and strives to comply with the Accreditation Council for Continuing Medical Education (ACCME) Standards of Commercial Support, Commonwealth of Virginia statutes, University of Virginia policies and procedures, and associated federal and private regulations and guidelines on the need for disclosure and monitoring of proprietary and financial interests that may affect the scientific integrity and balance of content delivered in continuing medical education activities under our auspices.

The University of Virginia School of Medicine requires that all CME activities accredited through this institution be developed independently and be scientifically rigorous, balanced and objective in the presentation/discussion of its content, theories and practices.

All authors/editors participating in an accredited CME activity are expected to disclose to the readers relevant financial relationships with commercial entities occurring within the past 12 months (such as grants or research support, employee, consultant, stock holder, member of speakers bureau, etc.). The University of Virginia School of Medicine will employ appropriate mechanisms to resolve potential conflicts of interest to maintain the standards of fair and balanced education to the reader. Questions about specific strategies can be directed to the Office of Continuing Medical Education, University of Virginia School of Medicine, Charlottesville, Virginia.

The authors/editors listed below have identified no professional or financial affiliations for themselves or their spouse/partner:

Stacy Ackerlind, PhD; Joseph F. Audette, MD; Nasr Enany, MD; Rachel Glover (Acquisitions Editor); Steven H. Horowitz, MD; Helena Knotgova, PhD; Gary McCleane, MD; Jim McLean, MD; Muhammad A. Munir, MD; Marco Pappagallo, MD; Gira Patel, L.Ac.; Lynn R. Rader, MD; Howard S. Smith, MD (Guest Editor); Robert Teasell, MD; Todd W. Vanderah, MD; and, Jun-Ming Zhang, MSc, MD.

The authors/editors listed below identified the following professional or financial affiliations for themselves or their spouse/partner:

David Euler, L.Ac. owns stock in Kiiko Matsumoto International.
Harold Merskey, DM, FRCPC is on the advisory committee for Fralex Therapeutics; and owns stock in Pfizer and Merck.
Akiko Okifuji, PhD is on the speaker's bureau for Janssen.
Steven P. Stanos, DO is on the speaker's bureau for Pfizer, PriCara, and Cephalon; and is on the advisory board for Endo, Pfizer, Alpharma, and Cephalon.

Disclosure of Discussion of non-FDA approved uses for pharmaceutical products and/or medical devices:

The University of Virginia School of Medicine, as an ACCME provider, requires that all faculty presenters identify and disclose any "off label" uses for pharmaceutical and medical device products. The University of Virginia School of Medicine recommends that each physician fully review all the available data on new products or procedures prior to instituting them with patients.

TO ENROLL

To enroll in the Medical Clinics of North America Continuing Medical Education program, call customer service at 1-800-654-2452 or visit us online at http://www.theclinics.com/home/cme. The CME program is available to subscribers for an additional fee of USD 205.

FORTHCOMING ISSUES

RECENT ISSUES

GUEST EDITOR

HOWARD S. SMITH, MD, Director of Pain Management, Department of Anesthesiology, Albany Medical College, Albany, New York

CONTRIBUTORS

STACY ACKERLIND, PhD, Director of Assessment, Evaluation, and Research in Student Affairs, University of Utah, Salt Lake City, Utah

JOSEPH F. AUDETTE, MA, MD, Assistant Professor, Department of Physical Medicine and Rehabilitation, Harvard Medical School, Boston, Massachusetts

NASR ENANY, MD, Assistant Professor, Department of Anesthesiology, University of Cincinnati College of Medicine, Cincinnati, Ohio

DAVID EULER, LICAC, Course Co-Director, Harvard Medical School Continuing Medical Education Course, *Structural Acupuncture for Physicians,* Kiiko Matsumoto International, Newton, Massachusetts

STEVEN H. HOROWITZ, MD, Clinical Professor of Neurology, University of Vermont College of Medicine, Burlington, Vermont; Assistant in Neurology, Department of Neurology, Massachusetts General Hospital, Boston, Massachusetts

HELENA KNOTKOVA, PHD, Research Scientist, Department of Pain Medicine and Palliative Care, Beth Israel Medical Center, New York, New York

GARY McCLEANE, MD, FFARCSI, Consultant in Pain Management, Rampark Pain Centre, Lurgan, Northern Ireland, United Kingdom

JAMES McLEAN, MD, Pain Fellow, Department of Physical Medicine and Rehabilitation, Northwestern University Feinberg School of Medicine, Chicago, Illinois; Sports and Spine Rehabilitation Center, Rehabilitation Institute of Chicago, Chicago, Illinois

HAROLD MERSKEY, DM, FRCP, FRCPC, FRCPsych, Professor Emeritus of Psychiatry, London, Ontario, Canada

MUHAMMAD A. MUNIR, MD, Assistant Professor and Program Director of Pain Medicine, Department of Anesthesiology, University of Cincinnati College of Medicine, Cincinnati, Ohio

AKIKO OKIFUJI, PhD, Associate Professor of Anesthesiology, Pain Research and Management Center, University of Utah, Salt Lake City, Utah

MARCO PAPPAGALLO, MD, Director for Research, Department of Anesthesiology, Mount Sinai Hospital, New York, New York

GIRA PATEL, LICAC, Clinical Associate, Osher Integrative Care Center, Harvard Medical School, Osher Institute, Division for Research and Education in Complementary and Integrative Medicine, Boston, Massachusetts

LYNN RADER, MD, Clinical Instructor, Department of Physical Medicine and Rehabilitation, Northwestern University Feinberg School of Medicine, Chicago, Illinois; Attending Physician, Chronic Pain Care Center, Rehabilitation Institute of Chicago, Chicago, Illinois

STEVEN P. STANOS, DO, Clinical Instructor, Department of Physical Medicine and Rehabilitation, Northwestern University Feinberg School of Medicine, Chicago, Illinois; Medical Director, Chronic Pain Care Center, Rehabilitation Institute of Chicago, Chicago, Illinois

ROBERT W. TEASELL, MD, FRCPC, Chair/Chief, Department of Physical Medicine & Rehabilitation, University of Western Ontario, Parkwood Hospital, London, Ontario, Canada

TODD W. VANDERAH, PHD, Associate Professor, Departments of Pharmacology and Anesthesiology, University of Arizona College of Medicine, Tucson, Arizona

JUN-MING ZHANG, MSc, MD, Associate Professor and Director of Research, Department of Anesthesiology, University of Cincinnati College of Medicine, Cincinnati, Ohio

CONTENTS

each having pain-related symptoms and signs thought secondary to common pain mechanisms. Ancillary testing may demonstrate associated nervous system abnormalities, however its specificity is inadequate at present, as it makes inferential conclusions from indirect data. Symptom assessment and physical findings remain paramount in the diagnosis of neuropathic pain.

Social factors affecting estimates of pain severity are noted, including attitudes toward pain before anesthesia, changes in attitudes afterward, and roles of physicians as examiners for military service or for compensation. Physicians identified as experts by insurance companies may see patients' injuries as causing less discomfort than do those who work for patients. An example is provided of a report funded by an insurance influence. Two examples are provided of studies in which treatment of data was insurance-friendly. We emphasize the importance of recognizing social influences on the process through which compensation is determined. These influences may be adverse to the normal evaluation of pain even when compensation is not an issue, and efforts are required to minimize potential bias.

Pain is a complex, idiosyncratic experience. When pain is the primary complaint for seeking medical attention, understanding of multiple factors is essential in guiding successful treatment. Behavioral medicine, a branch of psychology, has been an integral part of interdisciplinary/multidisciplinay care of pain patients. In this article, we provide an overview of behavioral medicine approaches to pain, including assessment and commonly used therapeutic methods. Particular attention is given to cognitive-behavioral therapy and motivational enhancement therapy.

A physical medicine and rehabilitation approach to acute and chronic pain syndromes includes a wide spectrum of treatment focus. Management includes an assessment and treatment model based on a biopsychosocial approach. Assessment includes a focus on pain behaviors, posture, muscle imbalances, and gait impairments. Effective treatment programs rely on appropriate and realistic goal setting. Treatment options may include physical therapy, polypharmacy, cognitive behavioral therapy, and passive modalities. Treatment goals emphasize achieving analgesia, improving psychosocial functioning, and reintegration of recreational or leisure pursuits. More complicated multidimensional chronic pain conditions may require a more collaborative continuum of multidisciplinary and interdisciplinary treatment approaches. Progress in all therapies necessitates close monitoring by the health care provider and ongoing communication between members of the treatment team.

Nonopioid analgesics represent a varied collection of analgesic agents, many of which also possess antipyretic or anti-inflammatory actions. As a group, nonopioid analgesics represent reasonable first-line analgesics for a variety of mild to moderate painful conditions and also often may be useful in conjunction with other analgesics (eg, opioids) for a myriad of severe painful conditions. Clinicians treating pain should be familiar with the actions, adverse effects, and individual agents in the group of nonopioid analgesics.

Adjuvant analgesics represent a diverse group of drugs that were originally developed for a primary indication other than pain. Many of these medications are currently used to enhance analgesia under specific circumstances. The proper use of adjuvant drugs is one of the keys to success in effective pain management. Since adjuvant analgesics are typically administered to patients who take multiple medications, decisions regarding administration and dosage must be made with a clear understanding of the stage of the disease and the goals of care. The article discusses major classes of adjuvant analgesics, with the focus on the mechanism of action, clinical application, and risks and benefits associated with each particular class of adjuvants.

Historically, analgesics were applied by the topical route of administration. With the advent of oral formulations of drugs, topical application became less popular among physicians, although patients still rated this method of drug delivery as efficacious and practical. We now appreciate that peripheral mechanisms of actions of a variety of preparations rationalizes their topical application and gives further opportunity to target peripheral receptors and neural pathways that previously required systemic administration to achieve therapeutic effect. Therefore, a peripheral effect can be generated by using locally applied drug and, consequently, systemic concentrations of that drug may not reach the level at which systemic side effects can occur.

THE MEDICAL
CLINICS
OF NORTH AMERICA

Med Clin N Am 91 (2007) xi–xii

Preface

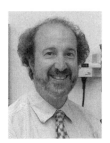

Howard S. Smith, MD
Guest Editor

Pain and suffering remain a significant dilemma. Pain continues to be among the most common reasons why patients seek medical attention (commonly for headache and back pain). Providing comfort and alleviation of pain and suffering remains a primary and crucial goal of patient care, as well as a great medical challenge. These issues of *Medical Clinics of North America*, *Pain Management* (Parts I and II), expose clinicians to a broad spectrum of available evaluation and management strategies.

The subjective nature of pain complaints, not uncommonly coupled with a lack of objective findings, continues to be troublesome for many clinicians who long for specific blood tests or imaging modalities that detect various pathophysiologies, in particular those which may help explain a patient's pain. Many physicians who are comfortable providing medical care to patients with hypertensive or diabetic issues do not have a similar level of comfort providing analgesia to patients with persistent noncancer pain.

In 2004, the American Society of Functional Neuroradiology (ASFNR) was founded to promote clinical applications of brain imaging techniques, such as magnetic resonance imaging (fMRI), positron emission tomography (PET), and an MRI method known as diffusion tensor imaging (DTI). It is hoped that these and other functional neuroradiologic techniques may eventually be clinically useful for patients suffering from pain and other symptoms.

In the Proceedings of the National Academy of Science (December 20, 2005), neuroscientists reported using fMRI to teach people with chronic

doi:10.1016/j.mcna.2006.11.001   *medical.theclinics.com*

pain to monitor and control their own brain activity (in specific regions)—
a high-tech version of biofeedback. Patients attempted to extinguish com-
puter-generated flames, and the intensity of the flames reflected MRI neural
activity in the patient's right anterior cingulated cortex (ACC)—a region implicated in pain perception. Patients who were best at quelling the flames
(neural activity in the ACC), reported the most pain improvement after
the session.

Using genetics in the assessment of pain and its treatment has only just
begun. Waxman's group at Yale identified the first inherited painful neuropathy from a mutation producing a hyperpolarizing shift in activation and
depolarizing shift in steady-state activation. Studies of families with autoso-
mal dominant erythromelalgia (characterized by severe burning pain
in the limbs in response to mild thermal stimuli or moderate exercise) have
demonstrated mutations in SCN9A, the gene that encodes sodium channel
Na(v)1.7 and which is selectively expressed within nociceptive dorsal root
ganglion and sympathetic ganglion neurons. Other genetic analgesic treatment strategies may involve selectively dampening the expression of undesirable genes using RNA interference technologies. Future work may enable
viral rectors to deliver small interfering (siRNA) molecules to reduce or
eliminate mRNA with resultant long-term suppression of algesia-promoting
molecules.

It seems that the analgesic magic bullet is nonexistent, and the list of
analgesic targets continues to grow. Future clinical analgesic strategies
may include investigator-driven preclinical strategies, such as modulation of
bidirectional communications between neurons and glia, ablation or inhibition of NK-1 expressing superficial dorsal horn cells, or intrathecal cytokine
therapy or proteosome-induced inhibition of ubiquitination pathways.

Despite the explosion of preclinical research, the art of clinical pain medicine remains in its infancy. Optimally, individually designed mechanistic-
based targeted analgesic treatments can be tailored for specific patients,
thereby eliminating or reducing pain to minimal levels. Although clinicians
remain limited in their ability to identify specific cellular/molecular mechanisms contributing to an individual patient's pain complaints, it is our hope
that these volumes will help clinicians approach the evaluation and management of patients with persistent pain.

Howard S. Smith, MD
Albany Medical College
Department of Anesthesiology
47 New Scotland Avenue, MC-131
Albany, New York 12208

E-mail address: SmithH@mail.amc.edu

THE MEDICAL
CLINICS
OF NORTH AMERICA

Med Clin N Am 91 (2007) 1–12

Pathophysiology of Pain

Todd W. Vanderah, PhD

*Departments of Pharmacology and Anesthesiology, University of Arizona,
College of Medicine, 1501 N. Campbell Avenue, Tucson, AZ 85724, USA*

Nature of pain

Pain is described as an unpleasant sensation associated with a specific part of the body [1]. It is produced by processes that either damage, or are capable of damaging, the tissues. Such damaging stimuli are called "noxious" and are detected by specific sensory receptors called "nociceptors" [2]. Nociceptors are identified as C-fibers and Aδ-fibers. By definition, nociceptors respond selectively to noxious stimuli. These nociceptors are free nerve endings with cell bodies in the dorsal root ganglia and terminate in the superficial layers of the dorsal horn of the spinal cord. Here they relay messages by releasing neurotransmitters such as glutamate [3], substance P, and calcitonin gene related peptide (CGRP) [4,5]. These "pain" neurotransmitters will result in the activation of the second-order neuron via their corresponding receptor. The second-order neuron crosses the spinal cord to the contralateral side and travels up the spinothalamic tract until it reaches the thalamus. From there the third-order neuron is activated, traveling from the thalamus to the somatosensory cortex, which allows for the perception of pain. It should be mentioned that at the level of the spinal cord, second-order neurons result in the direct activation of lower motor neurons in the ventral horn of the spinal cord, provoking a reflex withdrawal from the noxious stimulus. Likewise, there are interneurons at the level of the spinal cord that will modulate the incoming pain information.

Neural processing of pain signals

Several steps can be identified in the neural processing of noxious signals that can lead to the experience of pain.

Funding was provided by National Institutes of Health, National Institute on Drug Abuse grants R01 DA15205-01 and 02 PA-95-050.
  E-mail address: vanderah@u.arizona.edu

(1) **Transduction** is the process by which noxious stimuli are converted to electrical signals in the nociceptors. Unlike other sensory receptors, nociceptors are not specialized from the structural point of view (in contrast to, eg, Pacinian corpuscles or Merkel's disks), but rather exist as free nerve endings. Nociceptors readily respond to different noxious modalities such as thermal, mechanical or chemical stimuli, but *nociceptors do not respond to non-noxious stimuli.* Also in contrast to other types of sensory receptors, *nociceptors do not adapt.* That is, continued stimulation results in continuous or repetitive firing of the nociceptor and, in some cases, continued stimulation actually results in a decrease in the threshold at which the nociceptors respond (ie, sensitization of nociceptors) [6–8].

Nociceptive afferent fibers are typically pseudounipolar neurons, with a peripheral terminal and a central terminal. Neurotransmitters that are produced within the cell body (ie, in the dorsal root ganglia) are the same at both the central and peripheral ends of the nerve fiber. The neurotransmitters are released at both ends, participating in producing the pain signal peripherally, as well as in promoting events that lead to additional pain perception centrally. The release of neurotransmitters from the peripheral terminals of the afferent fibers is actually an "efferent" function of these afferent neurons. Peripheral release of neurotransmitter substances leads to the classic "axon reflex." This reflex leads to peripheral changes that are recognized as indicators of pain: redness, swelling, and tenderness [9].

The pain produced can result from *activation* of the peripheral nociceptors by the released neurotransmitters, as well as by decreases in the threshold of response of the nociceptive fiber and surrounding nociceptors (nociceptor *sensitization*). In addition, "sleeping" or "silent" nociceptors, which are normally not active, are recruited after tissue injury has occurred and can then respond to a variety of stimulus modalities [10,11]. Once activated, these previously silent nociceptors fire persistently. When nociceptors become sensitized, they respond to noxious stimuli more vigorously, ie, the same stimulus now produces more pain. This is called *hyperalgesia.* Curiously, normally nonnoxious stimuli can also produce pain, a phenomenon called "allodynia."

More importantly, opioid receptors located on the peripheral nerve endings, when activated by either endogenous or exogenous opioids (ie, administration of morphine), show inhibition of afferent firing. Morphine acting at mu opioid receptors (G-protein coupled receptors) results in the *indirect* opening of potassium channels. Potassium with its positive charge flows out of the nociceptor leaving the inside of the neuron more negative. The enhanced intracellular negative charge hyperpolarizes the nociceptor, resulting in a decrease in nociceptor activity (ie, analgesia).

(2) **Transmission** is the second stage of processing of noxious signals. Information from the periphery is relayed to the spinal cord, then to the thalamus, and finally to the cortex. Noxious information is relayed

mainly via two different types of primary afferent nociceptive neurons that conduct at different velocities.

C-fibers are nonmyelinated fibers that conduct in the range of 0.5 to 2 m/sec. Nociceptive C fibers transmit noxious information from a variety of modalities including mechanical, thermal, and chemical stimuli. For this reason, they are termed *C-polymodal nociceptors*.

A-delta fibers are thinly myelinated fibers that conduct in the range of 2 to 20 m/sec. All fibers respond to high-intensity mechanical stimulation and are therefore termed *high-threshold mechanoreceptors*. Some, but not all, A-delta fibers also respond to thermal stimuli; the latter are termed *mechanothermal receptors* [12].

These afferent fibers then synapse on a second-order neuron in the superficial layer of the spinal cord. This second-order neuron will send its axon across the midline and form the ascending spinothalamic tract that leads to the thalamus. It is in the thalamus that the second-order cell synapses with the third-order cell that projects to the sensory cortex.

The second-order cells in the spinal dorsal horn also have the capacity to change their response patterns in the circumstance of sustained discharge of afferent fibers (as would occur in the setting of an injury). Under these circumstances, these cells respond at lower thresholds and form inputs over a broader area in the periphery (ie, have expanded "receptive fields"). In other words, the second-order cells become "sensitized." This is termed "central sensitization" and also contributes to the phenomena of hyperalgesia and allodynia [13].

Once the nociceptive afferents have terminated in the dorsal horn of the spinal cord, they transmit the signal from the periphery by releasing specific neurotransmitters that are associated with pain. One of the most important neurotransmitters for pain and the primary afferent is glutamate, which can interact with both N-methyl-D-aspartate (NMDA)-type and non-NMDA excitatory amino acid receptors. Another important transmitter associated with the transmission of pain is an 11–amino acid peptide called substance P, which interacts with the tackykinin receptor family (G-protein coupled receptors).

(3) **Modulation** is a third and critically important aspect of the processing of noxious stimuli. This process represents changes that occur in the nervous system in response to noxious stimuli and allows noxious signals received at the dorsal horn of the spinal cord to be selectively *inhibited* so that the transmission of the signal to higher centers is modified. An endogenous pain modulation system consisting of well-defined *intermediate neurons* within the superficial layers of the spinal cord and *descending neural tracts* can inhibit transmission of the pain signal [14]. Endogenous and exogenous opioids can act on the presynaptic terminal of the primary afferent nociceptor via the mu opioid receptor by *indirectly* blocking voltage gated calcium channels as well as opening potassium channels. The inhibition of calcium

entry into the presynaptic terminal as well as the efflux of potassium (hyperpolarization) results in the inhibition of pain neurotransmitter release from the primary afferent fibers, hence analgesia. Opioids have a second site of action at the level of the spinal cord. Opioid receptors on the postsynaptic nerve (the second-order neuron), when activated by an opioid, *indirectly* open potassium channels resulting in hyperpolarization of the nerve.

Activation of the cortical descending neural system is thought to involve the supraspinal release of neurotransmitters including beta-endorphins and enkephalins [15]. These peptides represent two families of endogenous peptides that are believed to produce pain relief, mainly under situations of stress. This is critically important to you as a physician because when you relieve your patients' pain with narcotics, you are giving drugs that mimic the actions of these endogenous neurotransmitters.

(4) **Descending modulatory systems:** Activation of the descending system by endorphins occurs through specific receptors called "opioid receptors." These systems are activated in and around the periaqueductal gray (PAG) region of the midbrain. Such neurons then project to sites in the medullary reticular formation and the locus ceruleus (the major source of seratonin and norepinephrine cells in the brain, respectively) through uncertain circuitry (probably through disinhibition, that is, inhibition of a tonically active inhibitory interneuron). These descending fibers then project to the dorsal horn of the spinal cord along a tract called the dorsolateral funiculus (located in the dorsolateral portion of the spinal cord) to synapse with either the incoming primary afferent neuron, the second-order pain transmission neuron, or interneurons. These descending pain modulatory neurons either (1) release neurotransmitters in the spinal cord, especially serotonin (5HT) and norepinephrine (NE) or (2) activate small opioid-containing interneurons in the spinal dorsal horn to release opioid peptides (again through disinhibition). The released NE and 5HT act to (1) directly inhibit the release of pain transmitters from the incoming nociceptive afferent signal, and (2) to inhibit the second-order pain transmission cell. Activation of the descending pain modulatory system is a good example of why subjects report not feeling pain under conditions of stress, or perhaps other situations, where even though the pain is felt, the degree appears to be greatly modulated [16–18].

Summary of sites of opioid action: We can identify four sites where opioids can act to relieve pain. When you give morphine or other opiates to patients you are (1) activating the opioid receptors in the midbrain and "turning on" the descending systems (through disinhibition), (2) activating opioid receptors on the second-order pain transmission cells to prevent the ascending transmission of the pain signal, (3) activating opioid receptors at the central

terminals of C-fibers in the spinal cord, preventing the release of pain neurotransmitters, and (4) activating opioid receptors in the periphery to inhibit
the activation of the nociceptors as well as inhibit cells that may release inflammatory mediators.

Intracellular mechanisms of opioid analgesia

Recent cloning has identified three distinct genes,—one encoding for each of
the three (mu, delta, kappa) opioid receptors [19–22]. All three receptors belong
to the G-protein coupled receptor (GPCR) family. Agonist binding to opioid
receptors leads to a conformational change in the opioid receptor itself. This
conformational change results in the activation of an intracellular protein
called a G-protein. The G-protein is made up of three separate protein subunits
termed alpha, beta, and gamma. The alpha portion of the G-protein in an un-
activated state associates with guanosine diphosphate (GDP), hence earning
the name G-protein. Typically the alpha portion with its GDP will bind with
the beta and gamma subunits and exist as an intracellular trimeric protein. Although there are more than 100 different types of G-protein coupled receptors,
it is thought that the diversity of the G-protein subunit combinations offer diversity among agonist intracellular messages. When an opioid binds to an opioid receptor, the opioid-bound receptor undergoes a conformational change in
the receptor. This results in the exchange of the GDP for a guanosine triphos-
phate (GTP) on the Gα subunit. It is this exchange of GDP for GTP that activates the G-protein complex. Opioid receptors typically couple to a Gαi
subunit, and once the exchange of GDP for GTP has occurred, the αi subunit
will dissociate from the βγ subunit and inhibit the activity of adenylate cyclase,
a nearby membrane bound enzyme. Under resting conditions, adenylate
cyclase converts ATP into cAMP at some basal rate. cAMP acts as a second
messenger within the cell resulting in several events including the activation
of protein kinases and gene transcription proteins. Opioid receptor activation
by an opioid will result in the activation of the Gαi subunit and inhibit adenylate cyclase enzyme, hence significantly decreasing intracellular basal levels of
cAMP. This opioid via opioid receptor–induced decrease in cAMP indirectly
results in the inhibition of voltage dependent calcium channels on presynaptic
neurons. These voltage dependent calcium channels are important in the
release of neurotransmitter and transduction of neuronal communication. Opioid receptors located on the presynaptic terminals of the nociceptive C-fibers
and Aδ-fibers, when activated by an opioid agonist, will indirectly inhibit these
voltage dependent calcium channels via decreasing cAMP levels hence blocking
the release of pain neurotransmitters such as glutamate, substance P, and
CGRP from the nociceptive fibers resulting in analgesia.

In addition to the indirect inhibition of voltage-gated calcium channels by
opioid receptors, the βγ subunit of the G-protein will open inward rectifying
potassium (GIRK) channels allowing K^+ to flow down its concentration

gradient and out of the cell carrying its (+) charge. This results in a more negatively charged environment within the cell termed hyperpolarization. This opioid-induced hyperpolarization results in a decrease in cell excitability hence attenuating neuronal transmission [23].

Chronic pain

Chronic pain states, typically represented as inflammatory or neuropathic in origin, are characterized by enhanced perception of pain to a nociceptive stimulus (ie, hyperalgesia) and the novel perception of a normally innocuous stimulus as being painful (ie, allodynia). Our understanding of the mechanisms that drive these abnormal, enhanced pain states has grown considerably, and it is understood that chronic pain states depend in part on sensitization of the spinal cord, the activation of nociceptive pathways projecting to medullary and midbrain sites, and the activation of descending pain facilitatory systems. The latter appear to be essential in maintaining a sensitized state of the spinal cord.

Spinal sensitization has been thought to be a direct result of increased primary afferent discharges into the spinal cord that maintains a state of excitation. Injured nerves show spontaneous, ectopic discharges from injury-induced neuromas, and mechanical stimulation of the neuromas elicit sensations ranging from minor dysesthesias to intense pain [24–26]. Spontaneous ectopic discharge was generated in the dorsal root ganglion (DRG) of the injured nerves that remained after excision of the neuroma [27–29]. The generation of ectopic action potentials and spontaneous discharges from injured peripheral nerves increased within the immediate postinjury period and were maximal within 1 week of the injury, they declined very rapidly within 3 weeks, and were essentially lost within 10 weeks [30–32]. In contrast, behavioral manifestations of nerve injury endure for months after the initial injury [33–35]. Current evidence indicates that the initial discharges initiate a state of central sensitization, but neuroplastic changes within the central nervous system (CNS) maintain the long-term sensitized status of the spinal dorsal horn [33,36,37]. The neuroplastic activation of ascending and descending components of a pain facilitatory system is described.

Primary afferent inputs and spinal sensitization

The augmented primary afferent activity in the immediate aftermath of nerve injury produces a state similar to long-term potentiation, commonly referred to as spinal sensitization [38,39]. A specific type of sensitization may be suggested by the phenomenon of wind-up, which is observed as progressively increasing responses of spinal dorsal horn neurons following repetitive electrical stimulation of C-fibers [40,41]. This phenomenon implies that an initial stimulus produces sufficient excitation of post-synaptic cells and that these cells are not fully repolarized before the next stimulus arrives, and are thus primed to produce an enhanced response. Importantly, wind-up is nociceptive-specific [40–42]. The slow depolarizations of these dorsal horn neurons allow the development of temporal summation to inputs from primary afferent C-fibers, which may translate as increased pain [43,44].

These observations correlate well with studies performed with natural stimuli. Noxious stimuli applied to the skin enhance the excitability of dorsal horn units such that responses to subsequent stimuli are exaggerated, and repetitive C-fiber conditioning stimuli caused prolonged flexion reflexes in rats [44,45]. The persistent spontaneous afferent discharges after peripheral nerve injury are also believed to produce a similar sensitized state, leading to the enhanced pain observed in the neuropathic state [39,46–48].

Evidence for increased primary afferent activity is supported by microdialysis studies showing that the release of glutamate and aspartate from primary afferents is increased in response to intradermal capsaicin, formalin, or repeated electrical stimulation of C-fibers [49–51]. In a recent study employing microdialysis, it was found that spinal administration of NMDA elicited a long-lasting release of prostaglandin PGE2 and, subsequently, of excitatory amino acids. Spontaneous and stimulus-evoked release of substance P, CGRP, and glutamate from primary afferent terminals is increased after peripheral nerve injury [52–54]. The increased release of excitatory neurotransmitters from primary afferents, including glutamate, substance P, and CGRP, promotes the sensitization of target neurons and can lead to hyperalgesia by virtue of the enhanced responsiveness of the excited cell [55,56]. Primary afferent outflow is increased by glutamate acting at excitatory presynaptic NMDA autoreceptors on the primary afferent terminals [57,58]. This increase in primary afferent outflow amplifies the activity of the second-order neurons, which release nitric oxide (NO) and PGE2 that then promote further release of glutamate and excitatory neuropeptides from primary afferent terminals [59,60]. Taken together, these studies indicate that repeated or persistent noxious stimuli can cause the enhanced outflow of excitatory neurotransmitters that may interact and potentiate their excitatory functions, setting the stage for the development of central sensitization.

Descending pain facilitatory pathways maintain central sensitization

The rostral medial medulla (RVM) is considered to be the final common relay with respect to nociceptive processing and modulation, and receives inputs from the spinal dorsal horn as well as from the cortex [61–63]. The RVM's role in modulating a pain inhibitory system has long been recognized; it is now realized that the RVM also acts as a source of descending facilitation of nociceptive inputs at the level of the spinal dorsal horn [37,64–68]. Electrical stimulation applied in the nucleus raphe magnus of the RVM and surrounding tissue elicited excitatory responses in neurons of the spinal dorsal horns [69]. Although focal electrical stimulation of the RVM at high current intensities inhibits behavioral and electrophysiologic responses to nociceptive stimuli, stimulation at low intensities actually promote nociceptive responses [70,71]. Similarly, microinjection of glutamate, neurotensin, or cholecystokinin (CCK) into the RVM promotes a perceived noxious behavioral response [70–73]. Manipulations that attenuate RVM activity have blocked enhanced nociception caused by a variety of methods. Hyperalgesia induced by naloxone-precipitated withdrawal was blocked by the microinjection of lidocaine into the RVM [74]. Taken together, these observations indicate the existence of an endogenous pain facilitatory system that arises from the RVM [75].

Converging lines of evidence suggest that the development of abnormal pain states depend on the establishment of descending facilitatory mechanisms arising from the RVM. The application of a noxious thermal stimulus applied to the tail facilitated the hindpaw withdrawal reflex, increased electrical cell activity of the RVM, and was abolished by lidocaine microinjected into the RVM [76]. These results are consistent with the hypothesis that behavioral manifestations of chronic pain states is dependent on descending facilitation of spinal nociceptive input from the RVM since this region is a principal source of descending projections [61,66].

Considerable evidence now exists to show that the activation of descending facilitation from the RVM is essential to maintain the behavioral features of the neuropathic pain state [36,37,73,77,78]. Behavioral signs of neuropathic pain were blocked by lidocaine microinjected into the RVM [33,64,77,79,80]. The selective activation of on-cells with CCK microinjected into the RVM caused hypersensitivity to noxious and innocuous mechanical and thermal stimuli [81–83]. Electrophysiologic evidence strongly suggests that the population of RVM neurons that expresses the mu-opioid receptor is likely to drive descending facilitation [84–86]. The development and maintenance of neuropathic pain states may be linked to the increased expression or availability of CCK in the RVM.

Summary

The processing and interpretation of pain signals is a complex process that entails excitation of peripheral nerves, local interactions within the spinal dorsal horn, and the activation of ascending and descending circuits that comprise a loop from the spinal cord to supraspinal structures and finally exciting nociceptive inputs at the spinal level. Although the "circuits" described here appear to be part of normal pain processing, the system demonstrates a remarkable ability to undergo neuroplastic transformations when nociceptive inputs are extended over time, and such adaptations function as a pronociceptive positive feedback loop. Manipulations directed to disrupt any of the nodes of this pain facilitatory loop may effectively disrupt the maintenance of the sensitized pain state and diminish or abolish neuropathic pain. Understanding the ascending and descending pain facilitatory circuits may provide for the design of rational therapies that do not interfere with normal sensory processing.

References

[1] Melzack R, Katz J. Pain assessment in adult patients. In: Wall PD, Melzack R, editors. Textbook of pain. 5th edition. Edinburgh, UK: Elsevier Churchill Livingstone; 2006. p. 291–304.

[2] Sherington CS. The integrative action of the nervous system. New York: Scribner; 1906.

[3] Jeftinija S, Jeftinija K, Liu F, et al. Excitatory amino acids are released from rat primary afferent neurons in vitro. Neurosci Lett 1991;125:191–4.

[4] Lawson SN, Crepps BA, Perl ER. Relationship of substance p to afferent characteristics of dorsal root ganglion neurons in guinea-pigs. J Physiol 1997;505:177–91.

[5] Lawson SN, Crepps BA, Perl ER. Calcitonin gene related peptide immunoreactivity and afferent receptive properties of dorsal root ganglion neurons in guinea-pigs. J Physiol 2002; 540:989–1002.

[6] LaMotte RH, Thalhammer JG, Torebjork HE, et al. Peripheral neural mechanisms of cutaneous hyperalgesia following mild injury by heat. J Neurosci 1982;2:765–81.

[7] Meyer RA, Campbell JN. Myelinated nociceptive afferents account for the hyperalgesia that follows a burn to the hand. Science 1981;213:1527–9.

[8] Kilo S, Schmelz M, Koltzenburg M, et al. Different patterns of hyperalgesia induced by experimental inflammation in human skin. Brain 1994;117:385–96.

[9] Schmelz M, Petersen LJ. Neurogenic inflammation in human and rodent skin. News Physiol Sci 2001;16:33–7.

[10] Meyer RA, Davis KD, Cohen RH, et al. Mechanically insensitive afferents (MIAs) in cutaneous nerves of monkey. Brain Res 1991;561:252–61.

[11] Handwerker HO, Kilo S, Reeh PW. Unresponsive afferent nerve fibers in the sural nerve of the rat. J Physiol 1991;435:229–42.

[12] Meyer RA, Matthias R, Campbell JN, et al. Peripehral mechanisms of cutaneous nocicpetion. In: Wall PD, Melzack R, editors. Textbook of pain. 5th edition. Edinburgh, UK: Elsevier Churchill Livingstone; 2006. p. 3–34.

[13] LaMotte RH, Shain CN, Simmone DA, et al. Neurogenic hyperalgesia: psychophysical studies of underlying mechanisms. J Neurophysiol 1991;66:190–211.

[14] Yaksh TL. Central pharmacology of nociceptive transmission. In: Wall PD, Melzack R, editors. Textbook of Pain. 5th edition. Edinburgh, UK: Elsevier Churchill Livingston; 2006. p. 371–414.

[15] Fields HL, Levine JD. Placebo analgesia—a role for endorphins? Trends Neurosci 1984;7: 271–3.

[16] Mayer DJ, Price DD. Central nervous system mechanisms of analgesia. Pain 1976;2: 379–404.

[17] Boivie J, Meyerson BA. A correlative anatomical and clinical study of pain suppression by deep brain stimulation. Pain 1982;13:113–26.

[18] Fields HL, Heinricher MM, Mason P. Neurotransmitters in nociceptive modulatory circuits. Annu Rev Neurosci 1991;14:219–45.

[19] Evans CJ, Keith DE Jr, Morrison H, et al. Cloning of a delta opioid receptor by functional expression. Science 1992;258:1952–5.

[20] Kieffer B, Befort K, Gaveriaux-Ruff C, et al. The delta opioid receptor: isolation of a cDNA by expression cloning and pharmacological characterization. Proc Natl Acad Sci U S A 1992; 89:12048–52.

[21] Chen Y, Mestek A, Liu J, et al. Molecular cloning and functional expression of a mu-opioid receptor from rat brain. Mol Pharmacol 1993;44:8–12.

[22] Yasuda K, Raynor K, Kong H, et al. Cloning and functional comparison of kappa and delta opioid receptors from mouse brain. Proc Natl Acad Sci U S A 1993;90:6736–40.

[23] Jordan B, Devi LA. Molecular mechanisms of opioid receptor signal transduction. Br J Anaesth 1998;81:12–9.

[24] Devor M. Sensory basis of autotomy in rats [editorial]. Pain 1991;45:109–10.

[25] Wall PD, Gutnick M. Ongoing activity in peripheral nerves: the physiology and pharmacology of impulses originating from a neuroma. Exp Neurol 1974;43:580–93.

[26] Wall PD, Gutnick M. Properties of afferent nerve impulses originating from a neuroma. Nature 1974;248:740–3.

[27] Bennett GJ. An animal model of neuropathic pain: a review. Muscle Nerve 1993;16:1040–8.

[28] Kirk EJ. Impulses in dorsal spinal nerve rootlets in cats and rabbits arising from dorsal root ganglia isolated from the periphery. J Comp Neurol 1974;155:165–75.

[29] Koltzenburg M, Torebjork HE, Wahren LK. Nociceptor modulated central sensitization causes mechanical hyperalgesia in acute chemogenic and chronic neuropathic pain. Brain 1994;117(Pt 3):579–91.

[30] Han HC, Lee DH, Chung JM. Characteristics of ectopic discharges in a rat neuropathic pain model. Pain 2000;84:253–61.

[31] Liu CN, Wall PD, Ben-Dor E, et al. Tactile allodynia in the absence of C-fiber activation: altered firing properties of DRG neurons following spinal nerve injury. Pain 2000;85:503–21.

[32] Liu X, Eschenfelder S, Blenk KH, et al. Spontaneous activity of axotomized afferent neurons after L5 spinal nerve injury in rats. Pain 2000;84:309–18.

[33] Burgess SE, Gardell LR, Ossipov MH, et al. Time-dependent descending facilitation from the rostral ventromedial medulla maintains, but does not initiate, neuropathic pain. J Neurosci 2002;22:5129–36.

[34] Chaplan SR, Bach FW, Pogrel JW, et al. Quantitative assessment of tactile allodynia in the rat paw. J Neurosci Methods 1994;53:55–63.

[35] Malan TP, Ossipov MH, Gardell LR, et al. Extraterritorial neuropathic pain correlates with multisegmental elevation of spinal dynorphin in nerve-injured rats. Pain 2000;86:185–94.

[36] Heinricher MM, Pertovaara A, Ossipov MH. Descending modulation after injury. In: Dostrovsky DO, Carr DB, Koltzenburg M, editors. Proceedings of the 10th World Congress on Pain. Seattle: IASP Press; 2003. p. 251–60.

[37] Porreca F, Ossipov MH, Gebhart GF. Chronic pain and medullary descending facilitation. Trends Neurosci 2002;25:319–25.

[38] Ji RR, Kohno T, Moore KA, et al. Central sensitization and LTP: do pain and memory share similar mechanisms? Trends Neurosci 2003;26:696–705.

[39] Ma QP, Woolf CJ. Noxious stimuli induce an N-methyl-D-aspartate receptor-dependent hypersensitivity of the flexion withdrawal reflex to touch: implications for the treatment of mechanical allodynia. Pain 1995;61:383–90.

[40] Li J, Simone DA, Larson AA. Windup leads to characteristics of central sensitization. Pain 1999;79:75–82.

[41] Mendell LM. Physiological properties of unmyelinated fiber projection to the spinal cord. Exp Neurol 1966;16:316–32.

[42] Woolf CJ. Windup and central sensitization are not equivalent. Pain 1996;66:105–8.

[43] Ren K. Wind-up and the NMDA receptor: from animal studies to humans. Pain 1994;59:157–8.

[44] Woolf CJ, Thompson SW. The induction and maintenance of central sensitization is dependent on N-methyl-D-aspartic acid receptor activation: implications for the treatment of postinjury pain hypersensitivity states. Pain 1991;44:293–9.

[45] Woolf CJ. Evidence for a central component of post-injury pain hypersensitivity. Nature 1983;306:686–8.

[46] Woolf CJ, Wiesenfeld-Hallin Z. The systemic administration of local anaesthetics produces a selective depression of C-afferent fibre evoked activity in the spinal cord. Pain 1985;23: 361–74.

[47] Ziegler EA, Magerl W, Meyer RA, et al. Secondary hyperalgesia to punctate mechanical stimuli. Central sensitization to A-fibre nociceptor input. Brain 1999;122(Pt 12):2245–57.

[48] Zimmermann M. Pathobiology of neuropathic pain. Eur J Pharmacol 2001;429:23–37.

[49] Paleckova V, Palecek J, McAdoo DJ, et al. The non-NMDA antagonist CNQX prevents release of amino acids into the rat spinal cord dorsal horn evoked by sciatic nerve stimulation. Neurosci Lett 1992;148:19–22.

[50] Skilling SR, Smullin DH, Beitz AJ, et al. Extracellular amino acid concentrations in the dorsal spinal cord of freely moving rats following veratridine and nociceptive stimulation. J Neurochem 1988;51:127–32.

[51] Sluka KA, Willis WD. Increased spinal release of excitatory amino acids following intradermal injection of capsaicin is reduced by a protein kinase G inhibitor. Brain Res 1998;798: 281–6.

[52] Koetzner L, Hua XY, Lai J, et al. Nonopioid actions of intrathecal dynorphin evoke spinal excitatory amino acid and prostaglandin E2 release mediated by cyclooxygenase-1 and -2. J Neurosci 2004;24:1451–8.

[53] Gardell LR, Vanderah TW, Gardell SE, et al. Enhanced evoked excitatory transmitter release in experimental neuropathy requires descending facilitation. J Neurosci 2003;23: 8370–9.

[54] Wallin J, Schott E. Substance P release in the spinal dorsal horn following peripheral nerve injury. Neuropeptides 2002;36:252–6.

[55] Ma QP, Woolf CJ. Involvement of neurokinin receptors in the induction but not the maintenance of mechanical allodynia in rat flexor motoneurones. J Physiol 1995;486: 769–77.

[56] Sun R-Q, Lawand NB, Lin Q, et al. Role of calcitonin gene-related peptide in the sensitization of dorsal horn neurons to mechanical stimulation after intradermal injection of capsaicin. J Neurophysiol 2004;92:320–6.

[57] Liu H, Wang H, Sheng M, et al. Evidence for presynaptic N-methyl-D-aspartate autoreceptors in the spinal cord dorsal horn. Proc Natl Acad Sci U S A 1994;91:8383–7.

[58] Ohishi H, Nomura S, Ding YQ, et al. Presynaptic localization of a metabotropic glutamate receptor, mGluR7, in the primary afferent neurons: an immunohistochemical study in the rat. Neurosci Lett 1995;202:85–8.

[59] Kawamata T, Omote K. Activation of spinal N-methyl-D-aspartate receptors stimulates a nitric oxide/cyclic guanosine 3,5-monophosphate/glutamate release cascade in nociceptive signaling. Anesthesiology 1999;91:1415–24.

[60] Liu H, Mantyh PW, Basbaum AI. NMDA-receptor regulation of substance P release from primary afferent nociceptors. Nature 1997;386:721–4.

[61] Fields HL, Basbaum AI. Central nervous system mechanisms of pain modulation. In: Wall PD, Melzack R, editors. Textbook of pain. 4th edition. Edinburgh, UK: Churchill Livingstone; 1999. p. 309–29.

[62] Fields HL, Bry J, Hentall I, et al. The activity of neurons in the rostral medulla of the rat during withdrawal from noxious heat. J Neurosci 1983;3:2545–52.

[63] Fields HL, Heinricher MM. Anatomy and physiology of a nociceptive modulatory system. Philos Trans R Soc Lond B Biol Sci 1985;308:361–74.

[64] Calejesan AA, Kim SJ, Zhuo M. Descending facilitatory modulation of a behavioral nociceptive response by stimulation in the adult rat anterior cingulate cortex. Eur J Pain 2000; 4:83–96.

[65] Fields HL. Is there a facilitating component to central pain modulation? APS Journal 1992; 1:71–8.

[66] Gebhart GF. Descending modulation of pain. Neurosci Biobehav Rev 2004;27:729–37.

[67] Urban MO, Gebhart GF. Supraspinal contributions to hyperalgesia. Proc Natl Acad Sci U S A 1999;96:7687–92.

[68] Zhuo M, Gebhart GF. Biphasic modulation of spinal nociceptive transmission from the medullary raphe nuclei in the rat. J Neurophysiol 1997;78:746–58.

[69] Cervero F, Wolstencroft JH. A positive feedback loop between spinal cord nociceptive pathways and antinociceptive areas of the cat's brain stem. Pain 1984;20:125–38.

[70] Zhuo M, Gebhart GF. Characterization of descending inhibition and facilitation from the nuclei reticularis gigantocellularis and gigantocellularis pars alpha in the rat. Pain 1990; 42:337–50.

[71] Zhuo M, Gebhart GF. Characterization of descending facilitation and inhibition of spinal nociceptive transmission from the nuclei reticularis gigantocellularis and gigantocellularis pars alpha in the rat. J Neurophysiol 1992;67:1599–614.

[72] Urban MO, Zahn PK, Gebhart GF. Descending facilitatory influences from the rostral medial medulla mediate secondary, but not primary hyperalgesia in the rat. Neuroscience 1999; 90:349–52.

[73] Xie YY, Herman DS, Stiller C-O, et al. Mediation of opioid-induced paradoxical pain and antinociceptive tolerance by cholecystokinin in the rostral ventromedial medulla. J Neurosci 2005;25(2):409–16.

[74] Kaplan H, Fields HL. Hyperalgesia during acute opioid abstinence: evidence for a nociceptive facilitating function of the rostral ventromedial medulla. J Neurosci 1991;11:1433–9.

[75] Urban MO, Gebhart GF. Characterization of biphasic modulation of spinal nociceptive transmission by neurotensin in the rat rostral ventromedial medulla. J Neurophysiol 1997; 78:1550–62.

[76] Morgan MM, Fields HL. Pronounced changes in the activity of nociceptive modulatory neurons in the rostral ventromedial medulla in response to prolonged thermal noxious stimuli. J Neurophysiol 1994;72:1161–70.

[77] Vanderah TW, Suenaga NMH, Ossipov MH, et al. Tonic descending facilitation from the rostral ventromedial medulla mediates opioid-induced abnormal pain and antinociceptive tolerance. J Neurosci 2001;21(1):279–86.

[78] Ossipov MH, Lai J, Malan TP Jr, et al. Tonic descending facilitation as a mechanism of neuropathic pain. In: Hansson PT, Fields HL, Hill RG, et al, editors. Neuropatic pain: pathophysiology and treatment. Seattle: IASP Press; 2001. p. 107–24.

[79] Mansikka H, Pertovaara A. Supraspinal influence on hindlimb withdrawal thresholds and mustard oil-induced secondary allodynia in rats. Brain Res Bull 1997;42:359–65.

[80] Pertovaara A, Wei H, Hamalainen MM. Lidocaine in the rostroventromedial medulla and the periaqueductal gray attenuates allodynia in neuropathic rats. Neurosci Lett 1996;218: 127–30.

[81] Heinricher MM, Neubert MJ. Neural basis for the hyperalgesic action of cholecystokinin in the rostral ventromedial medulla. J Neurophysiol 2004;92:1982–9.

[82] Kovelowski CJ, Ossipov MH, Sun H, et al. Supraspinal cholecystokinin may drive tonic descending facilitation mechanisms to maintain neuropathic pain in the rat. Pain 2000;87: 265–73.

[83] Friedrich AE, Gebhart GF. Modulation of visceral hyperalgesia by morphine and cholecystokinin from the rat rostroventral medial medulla. Pain 2003;104(1–2):93–101.

[84] Heinricher MM, Morgan MM, Fields HL. Direct and indirect actions of morphine on medullary neurons that modulate nociception. Neuroscience 1992;48:533–43.

[85] Heinricher MM, Morgan MM, Tortorici V, et al. Disinhibition of off-cells and antinociception produced by an opioid action within the rostral ventromedial medulla. Neuroscience 1994;63:279–88.

[86] Pan ZZ, Williams JT, Osborne PB. Opioid actions on single nucleus raphe magnus neurons from rat and guinea-pig in vitro. J Physiol 1990;427:519–32.

ELSEVIER
SAUNDERS

Med Clin N Am 91 (2007) 13–20

THE MEDICAL
CLINICS
OF NORTH AMERICA

The Taxonomy of Pain

Harold Merskey, DM, FRCP, FRCPC, FRCPsych

71 Logan Avenue, London, Ontario N5Y 2P9, Canada

Taxonomy is the theory and practice of classification. For an ideal classification each item to be considered should be independent of all other items so that it stands in its own place in the classification. For example, if we wish to classify peoples' names for a telephone directory, each name must represent a separate and distinguishable item. The classification must also be comprehensive. If two or more people have names such as John A. Smith then an additional criterion must be used to distinguish each John A. Smith and that can be done by adding a street address. If there are two John A. Smiths, each with his own telephone number at exactly the same address—most likely father and son, or if there are three, grandfather, father, and son—they may use a numerical superscript or a numerical postscript as John A. Smith[1], John A. Smith[2], John A. Smith[3]. That provides a perfect classification useful for the purpose for which it is intended, and of little or no interest besides.

Natural classifications such as animal, vegetable, or mineral are more exciting and even sometimes intellectually beautiful, for example, the periodic table in chemistry. Nearly always (apart perhaps from some isotopes made by humans) this meets the highest standards of classification also. Each element has a place of its own into which it fits and no other element with which it can be confused. Evolutionary classifications of flora and fauna similarly achieve great success although disputes may arise in marginal cases.

Medical classification lacks the rigor either of the telephone directory or the periodic table. It is exceptionally untidy but it is taken to reflect in some way "the absolute truth" or at least the wonderful truth as known to the best practitioners. Accordingly, physicians endeavor to create true descriptions of individual "true" disorders, each helping to some extent to improve upon the worth of the previous ones. Classification may then be bedeviled by an argument about the criteria that apply to a particular diagnosis, eg,

E-mail address: harold.merskey@sympatico.ca

what *is* Cervicogenic Headache? What *is* the difference after an injury between that and Migraine if Migraine occurs with photophobia or phonophobia and nausea? Are there two or more disorders each with its essential characteristics?

These disputes form an interesting adjunct to classification and may or may not be illuminating but resolving them is not part of the primary function of a classificatory system. Classification is not a means of reaching an absolute truth but rather a means of establishing ways to code data that can be shared and compared between different practitioners or investigators.

The main task of the classifier is simply to make sure that individuals can identify and locate types of object or events. The classifier is not required to establish a true "meaning" [1]. Thus, if physicians in different parts of the world wish to exchange information about headache it is not necessarily important to resolve first whether migraine should or should not include phonophobia in its classification. Rather it is important to identify headaches that are unilateral or bilateral, and then whether photophobia, phonophobia, nausea, and vomiting occur together with varying durations of the event. Thus, data can be collected for comparison between different groups with respect to the items used to identify particular events and any consequences that we wish to suppose follow from them, such as loss of response to different treatments and so forth. Of course, this does mean that one has to have some sort of idea about which criteria one wishes to put together in one classificatory slot and which criteria go into another classificatory slot. We are not really interested in comparing cases of headache with cases of elephantiasis. That separation is easily made. Separations between types of headache become a topic for study within the framework of an overall definition.

It is just as well that classification can be used in the way just mentioned. Were that not the case we would be left with irreconcilable arguments and spend all our time trying to determine whether all physical illnesses were hereditary and secondary to psychological status, or whether some physical illnesses certainly were due to environmental causes and others resulted from ill treatment in childhood.

A workable system of classification needs to proceed on the basis of information that is largely agreed and to define areas of disagreement so that they can be further explored. This is a reasonable way to avoid controversy about medical diagnoses and to pursue knowledge.

Existing medical classifications

Existing medical classifications vary enormously but are all, or nearly all, illogical. In the ICD-10 [2] for example we find that conditions are classified by causal agent, eg, infectious diseases or neoplasms; by systems of the body, eg, gastrointestinal or genito-urinary; or by symptom pattern and type of psychiatric illnesses, which include affective psychosis, schizophrenic psychosis, organic psychoses, depressive and anxiety disorders, and personality disorders.

All of the psychiatric conditions just mentioned, except for Personality Disorders, are segregated into a category known in the American Psychiatric Association's *Diagnostic and Statistical Manual* in several editions (DSM-IV TR at present [3]) as "Axis I Type Disorders" and Personality Disorders are classified in an additional Axis (Axis II). Patients may have any number of disorders from Axis I, eg, Major Depressive Disorder plus Post-Traumatic Stress Disorder, and another diagnosis as well on Axis II, eg, 301.4 Obsessive Compulsive Personality Disorder.

Medical diagnoses can also be classified by time of occurrence in relation to stages of life, for instance, congenital anomalies, conditions originating in the perinatal period, or presenile and senile disorders. At the lowest level of classification, ie, the simplest and least complex description of phenomena, conditions used to be classified simply as "Symptoms, Signs and Ill-Defined Conditions" and now as Symptoms and Signs, which actually constitute a group on their own in the ICD-10 [2]. Not only illness is classified in medical lists. There was also a code in ICD-9 [4], ICD650, for delivery in a completely normal case of pregnancy. The nearest to this now appears in ICD-10 as Single Spontaneous Delivery.

Within the major medical groups of ICD-9 and -10 and particularly the neurological section, there are subdivisions by symptom pattern such as epilepsy or migraine, by the presence of hereditary or degenerative disease, eg, cerebral degenerations that may be manifest in childhood or adult life, and by symptom pattern, eg, Parkinson's disease, Chorea, and types of cellular change.

Accordingly, there are also diagnoses by location, for example, spinocerebellar disease and by infectious causes within the neurological group (which is defined first by location, for example, meningitis).

If we look at pain disorders there are codes in the ICD-10 for Migraine (G43) and nine subtypes, and separately for "Other Headache Syndromes" (G44) with 10 subcategories. For Juvenile Ankylosing Spondylitis (MO81), and for Ankylosing Spondylitis in adults (M45) as for Seropositive Rheumatoid Arthritis (M05) with six subordinate categories and for Other Rheumatoid Arthritis with nine subordinate categories (MO6). Among Symptoms and Signs we find Headache (R51). The Cardiological section R07 includes precordial pain in the anterior chest wall (NOS) and this may be pain in the musculoskeletal system, or a neuralgic type of pain and precordial pain that may well not be cardiac. If we look at endocrinology we may simply diagnose diabetes, which was once one disorder but is now defined in terms of five subtypes on a biochemical and therapeutic basis, while among musculoskeletal conditions we have fibromyalgia defined by a distribution of pain and tender points and not by what might be its supposed innermost essence, while repetitive strain syndrome is diagnosed, whether rightly wrongly, on the basis of pain in parts that are overused.

To resolve some of the problems of comparing these illnesses, the American Psychiatric Association's *Diagnostic and Statistical Manual,* third edition [5], provided at least five different Axes on which conditions might be classified including Axis I—Clinical Syndromes, Axis II—Personality Disorders, or Specific Development Disorders, Axis III—Physical Disorders and Conditions, Axis IV—Severity of Psycho-Social Stressors, and Axis V—the Highest Level of Adaptive Functioning in the Past Year. This system allows us to classify both symptom patterns and also people, an interesting conclusion although the classification of people is notoriously unreliable whether by psychiatrists or anyone else in the medical context.

To add to these hazards we can also note that we may diagnose in psychiatric conditions from genetics, eg, Huntington's Chorea, symptom pattern, eg, schizophrenia, depression, bipolar illness, reported mechanism (tension headache), and even the presence or absence of irrational behavior, ie, psychosis versus neurosis, although the latter term is not much used nowadays, and was dropped from the third edition of DSM-III onwards.

One of the obvious responses in a situation where classification cannot be provided on a theoretical basis is to provide agreed operational definitions. This brings us back to the starting point of this discussion where it was pointed out that only two things really matter in a classification system, one is a distinction between A, B, and C and the other is that everything from A to Z will be included that is part of the material to be classified.

It follows that even within medicine the range of classificatory systems can be enormous. There are highly specialized and valuable classifications that will code the varieties and degrees of a single diagnostic category such as stroke [6] and there are also classifications that cover not just the type of illness or condition examined but simply the reason for consultation. Thus the ICCPC, the International Classification of Conditions in Primary Care [7], does not classify diseases but rather the reason for contact between the family practitioner and his or her patient. Such a classification will include the reason for a patient being in the doctor's office, eg, advice on a symptom, review of treatment, completion of a referral form, completion of an insurance company form, and so forth. All these items are classifiable and can be examined for whatever statistical purpose desired. The one thing classification does not do is provide a statement of absolute truth about the ultimate meaning of all medical disorders—or even one.

Classification of pain

More than 20 years ago, citing others, it was said that, "There has long been a need for classification in the field of pain" [1]. A classification of pain was prepared originally for the International Association for the Study of Pain, and first published in 1986 [8] with a second edition in 1994. The aim of the classification is described in the introduction to the 1994 volume

[9] as being to classify the major causes of chronic pain and to organize descriptions of the syndromes.

At first it was not felt possible or desirable to classify all painful conditions. A good classification of pain was principally required for practitioners who were specializing in the treatment of painful disorders and who needed to distinguish them from other disorders and disabilities. Thus it was inappropriate to include the pain of appendicitis or tonsillectomy in a classification of chronic pain, but it was desirable to have a systematic arrangement of conditions that commonly caused chronic pain. Any attempt to do otherwise would of course have amounted to writing an extensive textbook of medicine. The purpose of such a classification would be to provide a means of communication between specialists in the field of pain, enable them to know that when one published a report on sprain injuries the same disorders in question would be at least broadly similar to that which a different person would call by the same name, even internationally. A few types of acute pain were admitted to the classification for comparative purposes and because they frequently gave rise to chronic pain, eg, post-herpetic neuralgia. The Taxonomy of Chronic Pain, which was produced by the Task Force on Taxonomy of the International Association for the Study of Pain (IASP), known at first as the Subcommittee on Taxonomy, thus attempted to cover the major causes of chronic pain and some illustrative examples of acute pain.

That being easily decided, the most difficult problem was to determine the best approach to organizing pain syndromes. It is obviously theoretically possible to arrange pain syndromes by region of the body, or by organ system, eg, cardiac pains, musculoskeletal pains, and pain due to neurological illness and so forth. One might alternatively arrange pain syndromes by their purported causes, eg, post-herpetic neuralgia, which is immediately obvious could also come under the neurological rubric.

The International Association for the Study of Pain classification

The Task Force on Taxonomy of the IASP decided after some vigorous discussion that it would be unwise to classify on the basis of etiology. Etiology is the topic that most concerns practitioners because we think that that leads us to make the most useful diagnoses. Diagnosis is seen as the avenue to correct treatment. To give up the idea that we can classify by etiology first means recognizing that the empirical methods of medicine are not yet good enough to provide etiological classification, at least in the field of pain.

An attempt was made by a group at the National Institutes for Dental Research in the late 1970s to classify orofacial pain by etiology. The IASP subcommittee concluded that although the classification was detailed and well worked out there was insufficient agreement on etiology to make that approach satisfactory for pain as a whole. An impressive classification had actually been developed by the late Dr John Bonica in his classic work *The Management of Pain* [10]. Bonica had started with regions of the body and only turned to diagnosis after he had arranged the subject by region. The committee was unanimous that the best way to start was by region of the body since this was the least controversial and should be the first basis for classification.

The next step was to look at whether systems, patterns of pain, or etiology should come next. Etiology again lost out. The system involved seemed to be the next obvious agreed basis for arranging observations on pain. Not only was etiology displaced from the first position and the second position, there was also agreement that it should be left to the end to work out what best we could about it. Accordingly, the next part of the classification system focused on the temporal characteristics of pain and the pattern of occurrence for which coding was provided. Everyone was comfortable after that in grading the pain according to its intensity and so the first four axes of a pain classification had emerged as regions, systems, temporal characteristics, and intensity combined with duration since onset. Finally, room was left for etiology and that was classified as genetic or congenital: trauma, surgery, infective or parasitic, inflammatory but with no known infective agent and immune reactions, neoplasm, toxic, metabolic, degenerative, dysfunctional (including psychophysiological), unknown or other, and last, psychological origins. Each of these codings acquired a number from 0 to 9.

As an example of how the coding system works consider common migraine. Migraine was coded 4 in the third axis on the basis of the pattern of occurrence being one of recurring irregularly. A period is inserted for convenience of citing extra numbers. Axis IV reflects the patient's statement of intensity and time since the onset of pain so that a mild pain present for 1 month or less was coded at .1, and a severe pain present for more than 6 months was coded at .9. Since this criterion can vary from case to case within the same diagnostic category, the letter X was placed to reflect the fourth axis, and to signify that each case would have its features determined on the occasion of coding, and not arbitrarily beforehand.

Code 7 concerning Migraine was a statement indicating modesty about knowledge of the exact origins of the condition. Thus the initially constructed code for Common Migraine ran 004.X7. However Classical Migraine also satisfies these criteria and therefore Classical Migraine was coded as 004.X7a and Common Migraine was coded as 004.X7b.

A code of 0 is given for the head, face, and mouth; 0 for the nervous system whether central, peripheral autonomic, or special senses.

As indicated the X code symbol was used to permit the clinician to determine the features of that particular case in accordance with whether the intensity was mild, medium, or severe, and the duration was less than 1 month, between 1 month and 6 months, or more than 6 months. Thus, mild intensity of more than 6 months was rated as 3, medium intensity of more than 6 months was rated as 6, severe intensity equal to or more than 1 month but less than 6 months was rated at 8, and so forth.

Last, as indicated, codes were given for etiology. Despite using five places organized at a default sequence of XXX.XX, which in the case of Common Migraine as just discussed, was shown as 004.X7b, a number of classifications could theoretically use these additional codes. To discriminate between conditions occupying the same five axis locations, additional letters were required, namely a, b, c, and d, so that Classical and Common Migraine were coded as 004.X7a and 004.X7b, respectively.

This system of coding by special characteristics is intended to allow comparisons between groups of cases. To the best of my knowledge it has not been used a lot in clinical practice or in research investigations. However, a number of the diagnostic categories have been popular, clinicians frequently referring to the descriptions and characteristics provided for them. This particularly applies to fibromyalgia and complex regional pain syndrome, conditions where there was more doubt about the traditional appreciation of the disorder. The section on Back Pain is also used by some. As well, occasional rare syndromes that appeared in the classification were conveniently identified through it by members of the IASP who were able to refer to relevant sections of the classification to assist a diagnosis. This was noted for example with the fairly rare syndrome of painful legs and moving toes, which sometimes also involves the arms and which is due to dorsal ganglion or spinal cord damage. This is a condition that was on occasion previously treated as "hysteria."

The use of classification

The uses of classification are thus essentially pragmatic. It is important to understand that issues as to what is a "real illness" or what constitutes "a genuine syndrome" are not easily solved and should not get in the way of the diagnosis and treatment of patients. Rather it is necessary to have a structured method of characterizing syndromes whether or not this describes their supposed true essence or is in accordance with particular claims about etiology or significance. Given the structured method we can proceed to identify the subordinate phenomena that may lead to a more refined diagnosis. Even when there is a refined diagnosis it still may not be something that can be called an absolute truth but rather a step on the way to improved management, which is what clinical medicine is actually about. Such a modest aim nevertheless does not inhibit clinical description from proceeding to more fundamental analyses by interested scientists who may or may not be the clinicians.

References

[1] Merskey H. Development of a universal language of pain syndromes. In: Bonica JJ, editor. Advances in pain research & therapy. New York: Raven Press; 1983. p. 37–52.

[2] World Health Organization. International classification of diseases and related health problems. 10th revision (ICD-10). Geneva: WHO; 1992.

[3] American Psychiatric Association. Diagnostic and statistical mannual. 4th edition (DSM-IV). Washington, DC: APA Press; 2000.

[4] World Health Organization. International classification of diseases and related health problems. 9th revision (ICD-9). Geneva: WHO; 1978.

[5] American Psychiatric Association. Diagnostic and statistical mannual. 3rd edition (DSM-III). Washington, DC: APA Press; 1980.

[6] Capildeo R, Haberman S, Rose FC. New classification of stroke. Preliminary communication. BMJ 1977;2:1578–80.

[7] Lamberts H, Wood M. International classification of primary care. Oxford: Oxford University Press; 1989 [Reprinted with corrections, 1989].

[8] Merskey H, editor. Classification of chronic pain: descriptions of chronic pain syndromes and definitions of pain terms. Monograph for Subcommittee on Taxonomy, International Association for the Study of Pain. Pain Suppl. 3. Amsterdam: Elsevier Science Publishers; 1986.

[9] Merskey H, Bogduk N, editors. Classification of chronic pain descriptions of chronic pain syndromes and definitions of pain terms. 2nd edition. Seattle (WA): International Association for the Study of Pain; 1994.

[10] Bonica JJ. The management of pain. Philadelphia: Lippincott; 1953.

THE MEDICAL
CLINICS
OF NORTH AMERICA

Med Clin N Am 91 (2007) 21–30

The Diagnostic Workup of Patients with Neuropathic Pain

Steven H. Horowitz, MD[a,b,*]

[a]University of Vermont College of Medicine, Burlington, VT 05405, USA
[b]Department of Neurology, Massachusetts General Hospital, 55 Fruit Street,
Boston, MA 02114, USA

Current concepts of acute and chronic pain disorders distinguish "nociceptive," "inflammatory," "functional," and "neuropathic" pains [1]. Nociceptive pain is the common pain experienced from trauma, cancer, and so forth in which pain receptors (nociceptors) are activated. Transduction, conduction, and transmission of nociceptor activity to a conscious level involves peripheral and central nervous system pain pathways, which, when intact, function in a protective and adaptive manner [1]. However, damage to, or dysfunction of, these pain pathways, peripherally or centrally, can result in a different, much less frequent, but nevertheless important pain picture—that of neuropathic pain.

Neuropathic pain is not a disease in and of itself, but rather a manifestation of multiple and varied disorders affecting the nervous system, particularly its somatosensory components. They include polyneuropathies such as those secondary to diabetes mellitus, alcoholism, and amyloidosis; idiopathic small-fiber neuropathy; hereditary neuropathies; mononeuropathies such as trigeminal, glossopharyngeal, and post-herpetic neuralgias; entrapment neuropathies; and traumatic nerve injuries producing complex regional pain syndrome (CRPS) type II. CRPS type I is also considered a neuropathic pain disorder, although evidence for nerve damage as the underlying mechanism is more controversial. Neuropathic pain can occur in central nervous system disorders, especially spinal cord injury, multiple sclerosis, and cerebrovascular lesions of the brainstem and thalamus. Neuropathic pain in these conditions confers no functional benefit and may be considered a "maladaptive" response of the nervous system to the primary pathology [1].

* Department of Neurology, Massachusetts General Hospital, 55 Fruit Street, Boston, MA 02114, USA.
   E-mail address: shhorowitz@partners.org

0025-7125/07/$ - see front matter © 2006 Elsevier Inc. All rights reserved.
doi:10.1016/j.mcna.2006.10.002   medical.theclinics.com

Unfortunately, the diagnosis of neuropathic pain is often problematic. Clinically, a distinction between nociceptive and neuropathic types of pain is not precise and conditions such as diabetes mellitus, cancer, and neurologic diseases with dystonia or spasticity can produce mixed pain pictures [2]. As with other pains, the perception of neuropathic pain is purely subjective, not easily described, nor directly measured. Also, pain pathway responses to damage are not static, but dynamic; signs and symptoms change with pathway activation and responsiveness, and with chronicity. Further, the multiplicity of disorders that have neuropathic pain as a component of their clinical presentations makes a single underlying pathophysiologic mechanism unlikely; more than one type of pain, and therefore probably more than one pain mechanism, can occur in a single patient, and some symptoms can be attributed to multiple mechanisms [2,3]. For these and other reasons the current management of neuropathic pain should be mechanistic in approach rather than disease-based [1]. Existing disease-based symptom palliation strategies should be supplemented with "targeted" mechanism-specific pharmacologic management [4].

History

Despite these complexities, there are several unique features to the clinical presentation of neuropathic pain that can be used to support its diagnosis and should be sought during history taking. In the case of mononeuropathies secondary to trauma, the severity of the pain often exceeds the severity of the inciting injury. CRPS can follow minor skin or joint trauma, bone fractures, or injections. The pain is stimulus-independent and described as "burning," "lancinating," "electric shock–like," "jabbing," or "cramping"; it is often accompanied by pins-and-needles sensations and sometimes by intractable itching (these are considered positive symptoms). These symptoms don't adhere to specific peripheral nerve distributions and often begin and remain most pronounced distally. The pain may be worse at night or during cold, damp weather, and is exacerbated by movement of the affected limb. Multiple types of pain (constant pain with paroxysms and stimulus-evoked pains) can be experienced simultaneously. It is useful to separate stimulus-independent and stimulus-evoked pains to differentiate ongoing from provoked activities [3]. Spread of symptoms outside the initial site of injury is common; in the case of unilateral pain there may be spread to homologous sites in the opposite limb (mirror pain). Positive and negative (numbness, loss of sensation) symptoms can occur concurrently and can be accompanied by autonomic symptoms. Spontaneous pain, often without complaints of sensory loss, is a feature of the cranial mononeuralgias—trigeminal, glossopharyngeal, and post-herpetic. Of course, location, intensity, and duration of pain are extremely important.

In generalized polyneuropathies, rapid progression solely affecting sensory fibers is more likely to be painful, especially if inflammation and ischemia are prominent pathological features, as occurs in the vasculitides [2]. In painful polyneuropathies, eg, idiopathic small-fiber neuropathy, diabetic polyneuropathy with predominant small-fiber (Aδ- and C-fibers) damage, the "burning," "lancinating," "jabbing" pains with pins-and-needles sensations are nerve-length dependent and bilaterally symmetric, beginning distally in the feet. With worsening, symptoms ascend to involve more proximal portions of the lower extremities and may eventually affect the hands. This centripetal progression can also occur in intercostal nerve distributions, beginning anteriorly over the midline of the torso with later symmetric lateral extension to the flanks. Autonomic complaints, eg, abnormal sweating, impotence, orthostatic hypotension, and gastrointestinal symptoms, are frequent.

Clinical examination

Among the more common and important clinical signs in neuropathic pain disorders are positive sensations: stimulus-evoked hypersensitivities such as allodynia to innocuous stimulation, eg, light touch and cold, and hyperalgesia to noxious stimulation, eg, pinprick. They occur focally in mononeuropathies and distally and symmetrically in polyneuropathies. Various forms of hyperalgesia have been described, including touch-evoked (or static) mechanical hyperalgesia to gentle pressure, pinprick hyperalgesia, blunt pressure hyperalgesia, and punctate hyperalgesia that increases with repetitive stimulation (windup-like pain) [2,3]. Paradoxically, these hypersensitivities can occur in areas in which the patient also complains of and demonstrates loss of sensation. There can be persistence of stimulus-evoked pain after the stimulus has been withdrawn (aftersensation) in the same anatomic distributions. As with symptoms, spread of allodynia and hyperalgesia outside the original site of injury is common and may extend to homologous sites in the opposite limb. Focal autonomic abnormalities after nerve injury, especially of sweating, skin temperature, and skin color, in conjunction with the aforementioned pain, fulfill the diagnostic criteria of CRPS (vide infra). With chronicity, trophic changes of the skin and nails develop, as do motor symptoms such as weakness, tremor, and dystonia. Nerve percussion at points of compression, entrapment, or irritation can elicit pins-and-needles or "electrical" sensations (Tinel's sign).

In small-fiber neuropathies, deficits are found in thermal and pain perceptions and sometimes touch, whereas large-fiber functions, eg, muscle strength, reflexes, and perception of vibratory and proprioceptive stimuli, are normal. In combined large- and small-fiber polyneuropathies, all these functions are compromised. Symmetrical distal autonomic dysfunction is often present but rarely severe.

While it is common for there to be relatively modest demonstrable clinical neurological deficits in patients with significant neuropathic pain, in some conditions there may be completely normal clinical examinations.

This is the rule in trigeminal and glossopharyngeal neuralgias and it occurs more than occasionally in post-herpetic neuralgia. But some patients, particularly with what appear to be small-fiber neuropathies or specific nerve injuries, who describe their pains with the aforementioned typical neuropathic pain adjectives, also have normal examinations. There is the temptation to attribute their pain complaints to functional etiologies; however, at least from a logical perspective, that cannot always be the case, and if they are known to have a particular disease such as diabetes, or suffered an injury in which nerve damage is likely, pain may be their only manifestation of neural dysfunction. In such situations and, of course, in most cases in which further diagnostic information would be helpful, ancillary testing can be used.

Ancillary tests

Any consideration of the utility of ancillary tests to support the diagnosis of specific neuropathic pain mechanisms must take into account several factors: (1) Currently, available tests only evaluate nervous system structures and functions presumed to be relevant to pain perception and transmission; from their results the presence, extent, and mechanisms of neuropathic pain are, at best, inferred. This situation is somewhat similar to testing for diabetes mellitus with peripheral nerve, ophthalmologic, and renal studies without the availability of plasma glucose levels. (2) There is a spectrum of clinical and physiological manifestations of neural injury within each disorder, with chronic pain occurring in only a small percentage of affected patients. For example, neuropathic pain occurs in ~16% of patients with diabetes mellitus and a third of those with diabetic neuropathy [5]; post-herpetic neuralgia, defined as chronic pain present 4 or more months after resolution of the acute herpes zoster (shingles) rash, occurs in 13% to 20% of patients [6]; and following direct nerve injury, as occurs during venipuncture, persistent pain is rare, perhaps occurring in 1:1,500,000 procedures [7]. (3) The causes of this clinical variability are less than certain, but the presence of pain is presumed to reflect damage to the small myelinated (Aδ-) and unmyelinated (C-) fibers within peripheral nerves [2]. As these fiber types also mediate other clinical functions that are measurable, eg, appreciation of painful stimuli, temperature perception, and autonomic activity, many tests have focused on demonstrating defects in these modalities to verify Aδ- or C-fiber damage.

Clinical neurophysiology

Neurophysiologic testing, principally nerve conduction studies and electromyography, are frequently used in suspected disorders of the peripheral nervous system. The usual techniques, with surface electrodes for nerve stimulation and evoked potential recording, measure activity of the largest and fastest conducting sensory and motor myelinated nerve fibers (Aαβ-). The most significant measured parameters are maximum conduction velocity (NCV) for the segment of nerve between the stimulating and recording electrodes, and amplitude and configuration of the resulting signals—the compound motor action potential (CMAP) evoked from motor fibers and the sensory nerve action potential (SNAP) evoked from sensory fibers. For central nervous system or proximal peripheral nerve disorders, somatosensory and magnetic evoked potential studies can be helpful. Electromyography (EMG) is the needle evaluation of muscles and evaluates muscle and motor nerve fiber activities.

Unfortunately, Aδ- and C-fiber activities cannot be tested with these techniques. Slowing in maximum NCVs or loss of CMAP or SNAP amplitudes, indicative of peripheral nerve disease either focally or generally, occur as a consequence of large fiber dysfunction. Abnormal EMG features such as acute and chronic denervation indicate involvement of large motor nerve fibers, also focally or generally, from the anterior horn cell distally. If present in a patient with neuropathic pain, these abnormalities can be used to corroborate the clinical impression of damage to a specific peripheral nerve or to peripheral nerves in general as in a polyneuropathy, eg, diabetic or alcoholic neuropathy. However, polyneuropathies or focal nerve lesions with only small-fiber involvement can have normal NCVs and EMG despite significant nerve damage and neuropathic pain.

Quantitative sensory testing

Quantitative sensory testing (QST) is used with increasing frequency, especially in clinical therapeutic trials, and measures sensory thresholds for pain, touch, vibration, and hot and cold temperature sensations. A number of devices are commercially available and range from handheld tools to sophisticated computerized equipment with complicated testing algorithms, standardization of stimulation and recording procedures, and comparisons to age- and gender-matched control values. With this technology, specific fiber functions can be assessed: Aδ-fibers with cold and cold-pain detection thresholds, C-fibers with heat and heat-pain detection thresholds, and large fiber (Aαβ-) functions with vibration detection thresholds. Elevated sensory thresholds correlate with sensory loss and lowered thresholds occur in allodynia and hyperalgesia [8]. In a generalized polyneuropathy when all quantitative sensory thresholds are elevated, it is inferred that all fiber types are affected, whereas if a dissociation exists wherein vibration thresholds are normal, but the other thresholds are elevated, the presence of a small-fiber neuropathy is suspected. In asymptomatic patients, abnormal QST thresholds suggest subclinical nerve damage.

The advantages of quantitation of sensory perception are that by enumerating an individual patient's findings and comparing them with normative values a clearer distinction between normal and abnormal responses occurs, thereby allowing analyses across patient and disease groups and for baseline standards in longitudinal studies. However, it must be appreciated that QST is a psychophysical test and therefore is dependent upon patient motivation, alertness, and concentration. Patients can willingly perform poorly, and even when not doing so there are large intra- and interindividual variations. Further, abnormal findings are not specific for peripheral nerve dysfunction; central nervous system disorders will also affect sensory thresholds.

Autonomic function testing

The evaluation of autonomic functions in patients suspected of having neuropathic pain can be important because of anatomic similarities between pain and autonomic fibers outside the central nervous system (CNS), and because disorders productive of neuropathic pain frequently have signs and symptoms of autonomic dysfunction (dry eyes or mouth, skin temperature and color changes, sweating abnormalities, orthostatic hypotension, heart rate responses to deep breathing, edema, and so forth). The majority of autonomic tests study skin temperature, and sudomotor, baroreceptor, vasomotor, and cardiovagal functions; they have been extensively reviewed [9,10]. A semiquantitative composite autonomic symptoms score (CASS), composed of the results of sudomotor, cardiovagal, and adrenergic testing, has been devised [11]. Less frequently, pupillary, gastrointestinal, and sexual function tests are helpful.

The value of autonomic testing in patients with a general neuropathic pain disorder, painful small-fiber neuropathy with burning feet, has been illustrated in several studies [12,13] in which many patients had normal or only mildly abnormal electrophysiologic (NCVs/EMG) findings. Autonomic abnormalities were seen in more than 90% of patients, the most useful tests being the quantitative sudomotor axon reflex test (QSART), thermoregulatory sweat test, heart rate responses to deep breathing, Valsalva ratio, and surface skin temperature [12,13]. However, in a recent study of patients with diabetic polyneuropathy, discordance was noted between efferent C-fiber responses in sudomotor tests (QSART and sweat imprint), and primary afferent (nociceptor) C-fiber axon-reflex flare responses. These findings indicate that these two C-fiber subclasses can be differentially affected in diabetic small fiber polyneuropathy. There may be involvement of one subclass and not the other or there may be different patterns of regeneration and reinnervation [14]. Autonomic functions can also be abnormal in peripheral neuropathies not associated with pain.

The relationship between autonomic dysfunction and pain is more complicated in CRPS in which focal sudomotor and vasomotor abnormalities are thought to be essential for the diagnosis [15] and sympathetic blockade has been a mainstay of diagnosis and therapy for decades. As would be expected, the vast majority of patients with CRPS were found to have autonomic abnormalities, particularly involving sweating and skin temperature [16]. However, there are patients with identical focal pain, but no clinical evidence of autonomic dysfunction. These patients do not meet the current definition of CRPS and have been termed "post-traumatic neuralgia" [17]; their autonomic functions have not been well studied.

Skin biopsy

For the past decade the histological study of unmyelinated nerve fibers in the skin has grown in importance in the diagnosis of peripheral nerve disorders, both generalized and focal, including those associated with neuropathic pain. When a skin punch biopsy is fixed with certain antibodies, most frequently protein gene product (PGP) 9.5, epidermal fibers can be stained and visualized [18,19]. Epidermal nerve fiber density and morphology, eg, tortuosity, complex ramifications, clustering, and axon swellings, can be quantified [18,19] and compared with control values [20]. A reduced density of epidermal nerve fibers is seen in small-fiber neuropathies [21], diabetic neuropathy, and impaired glucose tolerance neuropathy [22], each of which is associated with neuropathic pain. In a subgroup analysis of one such study, the skin biopsy findings were found to be a more sensitive measure than QSART or QST in diagnosing neuropathy in patients with burning feet and normal NCVs [23]. Conversely, disorders with severe loss of pain sensation such as congenital insensitivity to pain with anhidrosis (hereditary sensory and autonomic neuropathy IV; HSAN IV) and familial dysautonomia with sensory loss (Riley-Day; HSAN III) also have severe loss of epidermal fibers, as does a predominantly large fiber neuropathy, Friedreich's ataxia, in which pain is unusual [18,19]. Thus, the loss of epidermal small fibers is not specific for the presence of neuropathic pain.

Additional tests that may be of value in patients with neuropathic pain, particularly in focal pain syndromes such as CRPS, are bone scintigraphy, bone densitometry, and nerve or sympathetic ganglion blockade. Serum immunoelectrophoresis can be helpful in painful polyneuropathies associated with monoclonal gammopathies and acquired amyloid polyneuropathy. Specific serum antibody tests are valuable in painful neuropathies associated with neoplasia, celiac disease, and human immunodeficiency virus [24].

Summary

Determining the causes of neuropathic pain is more than an epistemological exercise. At its essence, it is a quest to delineate mechanisms of dysfunction through which treatment strategies can be created that are effective in reducing, ameliorating, or eliminating symptomatology. To date, predictors of which patients will develop neuropathic pain or who will respond to specific therapies are lacking, and present therapies have been developed mainly through trial and error [25]. Our current inability to make therapeutically meaningful decisions based on ancillary test data is illustrated by the following:

In a study specifically designed to assess the response of patients with painful distal sensory neuropathies to the 5% lidocaine patch, no relationship between treatment response and distal leg skin biopsy, QST, or sensory nerve conduction study results could be established [25]. From a mechanistic perspective, the hypothesis that the lidocaine patch would be most effective in patients with relatively intact epidermal innervation, whose neuropathic pain is presumed attributable to "irritable nociceptors," and least effective in patients with few surviving epidermal nociceptors, presumably with "deafferentation pain," was unproven [25]. The possible explanations are multiple and outside the scope of this review. However, these findings, coupled with the disparity in C-fiber subtype involvement in diabetic small-fiber neuropathy [14], and the recently reported inability of enzyme replacement therapy in Fabry disease to influence intraepidermal innervation density, while having mixed effects on cold and warm QST thresholds, and beneficial effects on sudomotor findings [26,27], when therapeutic benefit was demonstrated [27], lead one to conclude that the specificity of ancillary testing in neuropathic pain is inadequate at present, and reinforce the aforementioned caveats about inferential conclusions from indirect data. The diagnosis of neuropathic pain mechanisms is in its nascent stages and ancillary testing remains "subordinate," "subsidiary," and "auxiliary" as defined in Webster's Third New International Dictionary.

As a consequence of these difficulties, the recent approach by Bennett and his colleagues [28] may have merit. They have hypothesized (and provide data in support) that chronic pain can be more or less neuropathic on a spectrum between "likely," "possible," and "unlikely," based on patient responses on validated neuropathic pain symptom scales, when compared with specialist pain physician certainty of the presence of neuropathic pain on a 100-mm visual analog scale. The symptoms most associated with neuropathic pain were dysesthesias, evoked pain, paroxysmal pain, thermal pain, autonomic complaints, and descriptions of the pain as being sharp, hot, or cold, with high sensitivity. Higher scores for these symptoms correlated with greater clinician certainty of the presence of neuropathic pain mechanisms. Considering each individual patient's chronic pain as being somewhere on a continuum between "purely nociceptive" and "purely neuropathic" may have diagnostic and therapeutic relevance by enhancing specificity, but this requires clinical confirmation. Thus, symptom assessment remains indispensable in the evaluation of neuropathic pain, ancillary testing notwithstanding [28].

References

[1] Woolf CJ. Pain: moving from symptom control toward mechanism-specific pharmacologic management. Ann Intern Med 2004;140:441–51.

[2] Scadding JW, Koltzenburg M. Painful peripheral neuropathies. In: McMahon SB, Koltzenburg M, editors. Wall and Melzack's textbook of pain. 5th edition. Philadelphia (PA): Elsevier Churchill Livingstone; 2006. p. 973–99.

[3] Jensen TS, Baron R. Translation of symptoms and signs into mechanisms of neuropathic pain. Pain 2003;102:1–8.

[4] Smith HS, Sang CN. The evolving nature of neuropathic pain: individualizing treatment. Eur J Pain 2002;6(Suppl B):13–8.

[5] Daousi C, MacFarlane IA, Woodward A, et al. Chronic painful peripheral neuropathy in an urban community: a controlled comparison of people with and without diabetes. Diab Med 2004;21:976–82.

[6] Jung BF, Johnson RW, Griffin DRJ, et al. Risk factors for postherpetic neuralgia in patients with herpes zoster. Neurology 2004;62:1545–51.

[7] Newman BH. Venipuncture nerve injuries after whole-blood donation. Transfusion 2001;41:571.

[8] Suarez GA, Dyck PJ. Quantitative sensory assessment. In: Dyck PJ, Thomas PK, editors. Diabetic neuropathy. 2nd edition. Philadelphia (PA): Saunders; 1999. p. 151–69.

[9] Low PA, Mathias CJ. Quantitation of autonomic impairment. In: Dyck PJ, Thomas PK, editors. Peripheral neuropathy. 4th edition. Philadelphia (PA): Elsevier Saunders; 2005. p. 1103–33.

[10] Hilz MJ, Dutsch M. Quantitative studies of autonomic dysfunction. Muscle Nerve 2006;34: 6–20.

[11] Low PA. Composite autonomic scoring scale for laboratory quantification of generalized autonomic failure. Mayo Clin Proc 1993;68:748–52.

[12] Novak V, Freimer ML, Kissel JT, et al. Autonomic impairment in painful neuropathy. Neurol 2001;56:861–8.

[13] Low VA, Sandroni P, Fealey RD, et al. Detection of small-fiber neuropathy by sudomotor testing. Muscle Nerve 2006;34:57–61.

[14] Berghoff M, Kilo S, Hilz MJ, et al. Differential impairment of the sudomotor and nociceptor axon-reflex in diabetic peripheral neuropathy. Muscle Nerve 2006;33:494–9.

[15] Merskey H, Bogduk N. Classification of chronic pain: descriptions of chronic pain syndromes and definitions of pain terms. In: Merskey H, Bogduk N, editors. Task force on taxonomy of the International Association for the study of pain. Seattle (WA): IASP Press; 1994. p. 39–43.

[16] Chelimsky TC, Low PA, Naessens JM, et al. Value of autonomic testing in reflex sympathetic dystrophy. Mayo Clin Proc 1995;70:1029–40.

[17] Wasner G, Schattschneider J, Binder A, et al. Complex regional pain syndrome—diagnostic, mechanisms, CNS involvement and therapy. Spinal Cord 2003;41:61–75.

[18] Kennedy WR. Opportunities afforded by the study of unmyelinated nerves in skin and other organs. Muscle Nerve 2004;29:756–67.

[19] Kennedy WR, Wendelschafer-Crabb G, Polydefkis M, et al. Pathology and quantitation of cutaneous innervation. In: Dyck PJ, Thomas PK, editors. Peripheral neuropathy. 4th edition. Philadelphia (PA): Elsevier Saunders; 2005. p. 869–95.

[20] Umapathi T, Tan WL, Tan NCK, et al. Determinants of epidermal nerve fiber density in normal individuals. Muscle Nerve 2006;33:742–6.

[21] Holland NR, Stocks A, Hauer P, et al. Intraepidermal nerve fiber density in patients with painful sensory neuropathy. Neurol 1997;48:708–11.

[22] Polydefkis M, Griffin JW, McArthur J. New insights into diabetic polyneuropathy. JAMA 2003;290:1371–6.

[23] Periquet MI, Novak V, Callino MP, et al. Painful sensory neuropathy: prospective evaluation using skin biopsy. Neurol 1999;53:1641–7.

[24] Mendell JR, Sahenk Z. Painful sensory neuropathy. N Engl J Med 2003;348:1243–55.

[25] Herrmann DN, Pannoni V, Barbano RL, et al. Skin biopsy and quantitative sensory testing do not predict response to lidocaine patch in painful neuropathies. Muscle Nerve 2006;33: 42–8.

[26] Schiffmann R, Hauer P, Freeman B, et al. Enzyme replacement therapy and intraepidermal innervation density in Fabry disease. Muscle Nerve 2006;34:53–6.

[27] Schiffmann R, Floeter MK, Dambrosia JM, et al. Enzyme replacement therapy improves peripheral nerve and sweat function in Fabry disease. Muscle Nerve 2003;28:703–10.

[28] Bennett MI, Smith BH, Torrance N, et al. Can pain be more or less neuropathic? Comparison of symptom assessment tools with ratings of certainty by clinicians. Pain 2006;122: 289–94.

ELSEVIER
SAUNDERS

THE MEDICAL
CLINICS
OF NORTH AMERICA

Med Clin N Am 91 (2007) 31–43

Problems with Insurance-Based Research on Chronic Pain

Harold Merskey, DM, FRCP, FRCPC, FRCPsych[a],*,
Robert W. Teasell, MD, FRCP[b]

[a]71 Logan Avenue, London, Ontario N5Y 2P9, Canada
[b]Department of Physical Medicine and Rehabilitation, University of Western Ontario,
Parkwood Hospital, London, Ontario N6C 5J1, Canada

Diminishing pain

Apart from induced abortion there is perhaps no medical topic that causes so much dispute as the nature of chronic pain. The willingness to claim that chronic pain is "psychological" and therefore not as worthy as say, neuropathic pain, is a recurring issue in medical practice. The definition of pain published by the International Association for the Study of Pain (IASP) Task Force on Taxonomy is: "*An unpleasant sensory and emotional experience associated with actual or potential tissue damage or described in terms of such damage*" [1]. The original purpose of this definition was to provide a formula that covered all pain, whether it was thought to be a result of injury or a consequence of anxiety. Despite the apparent success of this definition many may fail to recognize that its original intent was to secure proper acceptance of the suffering of all patients with pain. Thus, a distinguished European author [2], recognizing the widespread acceptance of the definition, nevertheless emphasizes that this reflects "the first person perspective of pain" while for "*clinical neurology*" he says "third person perspectives are more important, because neurologists in their day-to-day practice deal with observable signs." This is a good example of how to accept something with one hand while rejecting it with the other. Many North American neurologists, and indeed others elsewhere, might disagree with the above statement, especially if their practice focuses on headaches with, mainly, no signs.

Declaration of interest: H.M. and R.W.T. both provide reports to lawyers concerning their patients and others, usually, but not invariably, for those seeking compensation.
* Corresponding author.
E-mail address: harold.merskey@sympatico.ca (H. Merskey).

Parallels are all too common, as Merskey and Spear [3] have shown. One example may suffice. Inman wrote in 1858, "In medicine pain is no pain and suffering no suffering, in an hysterical sense ... a hysterical pain is one which a patient feels but has not; which has no existence; but which, by being thought upon, may grow until it is unbearable" [4]. Loeser corrects these assumptions when he writes, "... Chronic pain can only be described as a set of behaviors. It has qualities that can be described: onset, duration, intensity, frequency, periodicity, quality. These behaviors can be measured also in terms of the amount of disability they produce...." [5].

It should not be necessary to argue that all pain meeting the definition deserves adequate proof. The challenge and the reward probably lie in elucidating the relatively amorphous pains of musculoskeletal disorder or fibromyalgia when compared with the more discrete effects of neuropathic pain.

These current citations affirm that misconceptions and honest questioning are both part of the current world of discussion of pain. In that discussion there is a constant hierarchy with respect to the value of different pains in which neuropathic pain trumps musculoskeletal pain, which trumps psychogenic pain. This is in part a natural attitude, a consequence of the difficulty in recognizing the unseen cause of another person's pain. Such a pain is less important to us than our own unseen experience or that of a beloved dependent. As well, the facts that the worst acute pains often have a visible organic component, eg, burns or fractures, leaves us wondering about the extent to which a seemingly undisturbed individual can be suffering from extremely severe chronic pain without much, or any, change in their countenance.

It was not always so. Historically pain was seen as a dreadful affliction whether acute of chronic [6,7]. Only after the development of increasing technical knowledge did changes in attitude occur. The success of anesthesia took away some of the fear of pain. The success of scientific medicine led to a neglect of the skills of personal relationships [8].

More than one factor may have contributed to an increasing under-estimation of patients' pain. At one time opioids were widely used and bought and sold in grocers' stores, both in North America and Britain. A reversal of opinion on the broad use of opioids developed during the nineteenth century. Physicians campaigned for recognition through licensure on the part of the state. In making this request they raised concern about the uncontrolled use of narcotics (which may well have been overstated) [9]. They succeeded in becoming responsible for restricting the chronic use of opium in return for formal recognition through licensure. In association with this responsibility their views on the use of opioids became more and more restrictive and pain seems to have become less and less severe in their estimation. If patients asked for too much opium and the physician gave in he would be breaking his undertaking to the State—and nowadays to licensing bodies—which have power over his ability to practice at all. The regulation of opioids thus created an instinctive bias on the part of physicians to question the validity of patients' claims of severe pain needing opioid relief.

Another factor emerged, particularly during the First World War, with respect to all types of medical complaint, not forgetting pain. Physicians on both sides became responsible for determining whether an individual was fit to return to battle. An illness that would take someone out of the firing line had to be proven. Subjective complaints without physical evidence were not accepted at face value. Physicians later also became responsible for recognizing patients' pain in another sense that is in connection with pensions. Again, there was pressure on the physician, although less severe in this instance, not to give way to individuals who might be overstating their case. The main factor working to correct an undue bias against the patient was the strength of the doctor's professional training. Sometimes rather than give in to the needs of the patient the physician chose to support the government, and later insurance companies. Among a plethora of potential psychological symptoms pain had one of the greater claims to organicity and one of the lesser claims to provability. In consequence, doctors began to see patients with pain, but without very strong physical signs, as less worthy than patients with independent evidence for their claims [10,11].

A further consideration has to do with compensation for workers and for others injured in industrial railway and other traffic accidents. One of the first, if not the first Act to provide compensation for injured workers was passed in Germany (originally in Prussia) to provide for railroad workers and miners [12]. A succession of Acts ensued in other countries in Europe and in the United States and Canada governing such situations. Physicians employed to work for the insurance industry tended to downplay the severity or intensity of patients' pain. The changes contributed to an emphasis on behavioral proof of the presence of pain. The consequence of this in clinical practice and in legal argument has generally been to emphasize that pain can be surmounted, and to disparage the pain of at least some individuals who were not able to overcome their pain by exercise. See for example, "Back Pain in the Workplace," a much criticized report produced by a Task Force of the International Association for the Study of Pain, which in effect recommended the abolition of compensation for back pain unless it was accompanied by strong supportive physical evidence so that if a sufficiently large lesion was not present in the MRI the patient should not be considered to have pain but after 6 weeks was to be described as "activity intolerant" [13].

After World War II a charismatic British neurologist, Professor Henry Miller, published an article that was highly influential, maintaining that injured claimants for headache followed up in insurance examinations all recovered once a verdict had been obtained [14]. This was not believed in the vicinity where he practiced (the counties of Northumberland and Durham, England) (Harold Merskey, DM, FRCP, FRCPC, FRCPsych, personal observation, 1957–1961) but it had a widespread effect from 1961 until 1982 when Mendelson [15] published an article entitled "Not Cured by a Verdict," which demonstrated that of 10 follow-up studies of compensable injuries published since the Second World War, not one supported Miller's conclusion and all agreed that pain persisted to a greater or lesser extent after legal settlement.

The theme of this article is that the view of pain may be diminished and minimized by members of the medical profession, sometimes directly because they have worked for insurance companies or provided opinions for insurance companies who seek such minimization of the suffering of their clients, our patients, and that such minimization of pain will extend not only to patients who have financial claims to make but inevitably to others who are being treated for pain by the same physicians. There is a natural tendency to seek consistency and it helps our conscience if we can say that we treat patients in practice for whom there is no insurance obligation in the same way as we treat them when there is an insurance obligation. That balance is somewhat more difficult to achieve in countries where medical care is provided through private insurers but the effect is evident even in countries such as Canada where the insurance comes from the government and, while not generous, at least provides physicians with their income without demanding that they satisfy any concerns the government may have over whether the pain that they are treating is disabling or not disabling [16]. Overall, however, in the article just cited we note widespread concern about the undertreatment of pain in many well-informed circles in the developed world. Claims to this effect have appeared in many places including the Royal College of Surgeons of England among others [17], but 14 years after a report of that body, pain assessment was still infrequently performed after operations [18].

Insurance-based studies

If the influence of working for insurance companies is worrying with respect to the impact it has on physicians' views of pain we should look carefully at relationships between the insurance industry and studies examining pain in insured persons. As a basic rule one might adopt the guidelines that are employed by pharmaceutical industries. We will discuss here guidelines for pharmaceutical companies in Canada but the principles must be closely similar to those employed in the United States. We have not encountered any specific guidelines issued by or to companies or physicians other than advice on how to write a medical report.

The basic guidelines of the pharmaceutical manufacturers of Canada relate to independent work that is funded by the pharmaceutical industry. Different considerations pertain to studies directly undertaken by employees or consultants of a pharmaceutical company. When a pharmaceutical company publishes information in its own name it is recognized that such material has to be understood as produced by the company in any case where it also appears to be beneficial to the company's financial interests. On the other hand, work that a pharmaceutical company funds by independent physicians and other practitioners is required to be funded through "an unrestricted grant" [19]. The topic may well be chosen in agreement and after discussion but once the grant is issued the conduct of the grant must be within the control of the investigator. Similarly with lectures, once an unrestricted grant is agreed for a lecturer, the content is entirely within his or her discretion. Clearly, this does not take away the existence of sympathy and willingness to be kind to the sponsor, but once agreement has been reached it does block the sponsor from attempting to have something changed that the sponsor dislikes no matter what the outcome of the actual study, or the way in which the lecture is delivered. Those rules appear to be capable of application to the insurance industry as will be seen shortly. Here, we look at one consensus statement and two studies that are known to have been funded by insurance companies. Those contributions to the literature were promoted by insurance interests and appear to lack the necessary restraint that should accompany the association of an industrial or commercial interest with medical conclusions.

Three publications

A Consensus Statement on Fibromyalgia

In 1994, the Physical Medicine Research Foundation organized a meeting in Vancouver to establish a Consensus Statement on Fibromyalgia. Among other conclusions this gathering approved a statement reached by a simple majority vote to the effect that fibromyalgia should not be diagnosed in the medico-legal situation. The statement had far-reaching effects. Fibromyalgia is a common disorder and commonly occurs in patients who have had chronic pain for some time. The pain generalizes and patients become extremely sensitive to touch. It is ordinarily managed by rheumatologists, and most of the physicians involved appear to have been rheumatologists. Until lately (M. Finch, personal communication, 2005) it was virtually impossible for a claim for fibromyalgia to be compensated in American courts. In Canada, it has been quite widely compensated although not so much in Alberta. The conference in question was attended by many prominent rheumatologists, presided over by a much-respected leader in the field, Dr Fred Wolfe [20]. Dr. Wolfe had however expressed concern about diagnosing fibromyalgia in individuals who might be compensated for it because of what he thought was the relative ease with which physicians might be misled. A number of rheumatologists disagreed with this position but the numbers of all those attending and voting at the meeting were not sufficient to prevent that particular line item being passed.

There was much discomfiture. Distinguished rheumatologists who had disagreed with the decision and felt that it was untoward and unfair to patients with fibromyalgia published an Alternative Consensus Statement also signed by others who were not rheumatologists but who had professional interests in fibromyalgia [21]. (As a pain specialist, H.M. was also a signatory to that second document although he had not attended the original meeting.) The alternative Consensus Statement rejected the view that fibromyalgia should not be diagnosed in circumstances where the possibility of compensation existed [21].

At the time of the meeting few knew about the background of the Physical Medicine Research Foundation. It was founded in 1982 as an "international" charity with American and Canadian contributions and a head office in Vancouver. It claims to be the first international charity devoted solely to funding research into chronic pain. It was little known to pain researchers before 1994. As clinicians actively involved in pain research and education we were not aware of it until we read about the meeting in Vancouver. At that time H.M. was chair of a task force in the International Association for the Study of Pain, dealing with classification, and a past president of the Canadian Pain Society. He often attended American Pain Society meetings besides. R.W.T. regularly attended Physical Medicine meetings. We had not encountered this body.

The Foundation had a very respectable international board of medical advisors, but it had no medical or health care board in Canada. Rather, it had two advisors in Canada, one in Vancouver for western Canada, and one for eastern Canada. Neither of those practitioners had specialist standing with the Royal College of Physicians and Surgeons of Canada (standing required for recognition as a specialist in an individual discipline). The board of the association was based in Vancouver and had 15 members of whom some 3 were linked with the insurance industry. More importantly, the Foundation had actually been founded by an industrial firm known as Woodbridge Industries with factories in 10 countries (and therefore injured workers in many countries), and two insurance companies, the Insurance Corporation of British Columbia (ICBC; a semi-independent organ of the provincial government of British Columbia) and State Farm, a very large insurance company operating in the United States and in many provinces in Canada. Most Canadian medical charities, we assume like American medical charities, have a medical advisory board made up of highly qualified individuals in the discipline with which they are connected. No such board existed for the Physical Medicine Research Foundation in Canada. Instead, there were the two individuals mentioned and a board, largely of lay composition in Vancouver, with one or two health care professionals. It was only in about 1996 approximately, that any person with Royal College qualifications (ie, Canadian Specialist Standing) in physical medicine and rehabilitation was appointed as an advisor to this charity [21]. The charity has subsequently changed its name, incidentally, to the Canadian Institute on the Relief of Pain and Disability, mimicking United States and Canadian national bodies with similar titles.

It seems the charity organized was heavily funded by State Farm and ICBC. Those attending the meeting who disagreed with the resolution concerning posttraumatic fibromyalgia recognized that many insurance personnel were present at the meeting.

It is hard to see the Physical Medicine Research Foundation, as it then was, and the meeting that it conducted, as being at arm's length from the insurance industry. It seemed in fact to those attending the meeting and who were uncomfortable with the decision that there were a great number of insurance personnel present and that they were quite concerned to establish a position about fibromyalgia that was not necessarily helpful to patients.

Issues connected with fibromyalgia and medico-legal argument have been prominent in both the United States and Canada in the existing literature at least for the past 15 years. The benefit to insurance companies of having a negative statement like that produced may amount to billions of dollars of compensation denied. Posttraumatic fibromyalgia accounts for 30% to 40% of cases in most reports [1,21] on the frequency of fibromyalgia. Compensation for individuals who are unable to work because of fibromyalgia, even in Canada where amounts awarded are relatively small, never reach the extreme size of those given in the United States, but may nevertheless reach figures approaching a million dollars. Given that fibromyalgia affects at least 3% or 4% of the general adult population and posttraumatic fibromyalgia represents say one third of those, we may suppose that at any one time there are 3,300,000 people with posttraumatic fibromyalgia among 330 million North Americans, putting the populations of Canada and the United States together. Even if just 100,000 people were to receive awards of $100,000 each, in a given year, for the effects of the pain and disability imposed by fibromyalgia on their lives, we could expect that at a conservative estimate a total of $10,000,000,000 could be reached annually. These figures are admittedly inaccurate and arbitrary but give some estimate of the scale of the savings that may have resulted to insurance companies from the denial of payments for fibromyalgia. Readers may ask themselves is it scientifically or professionally acceptable that insurance companies should have been so closely involved in the management of a medical meeting with such an outcome? There is at least fairly strong evidence to conclude that there was an unreasonably large involvement of the insurance industry's interest in the meeting.

A subsequent meeting, planned by the same body, was organized from February 7–11, 1999 with the following supporters: Platinum Sponsors: State Farm Insurance, Insurance Corporation of British Columbia, Workers' Compensation Board of British Columbia; Cash Prize Sponsor: Insurance Corporation of British Columbia; The Woodbridge Grants and Award Program: The Woodbridge Group, State Farm Insurance; Gold Sponsors: Manitoba Public Insurance, Motor Accidents Authority (Australia), Renault Car Corporation, Seaboard Life Insurance, The Woodbridge Group; and Educational Grants: Merck-Frosst. Merskey and Teasell commented at the time that "Such industry support is a double-edged sword.

Industry much more than government or charities, is likely to sponsor educational and research endeavors that help the bottom line. That in turn will influence which viewpoint is given greater prominence, particularly in whiplash where there is substantial controversy. This situation combined with a lack of strong scientific input, may account for BCWI's pattern of markedly downplaying the clinical significance of whiplash injuries" [22].

The Canadian Medical Association (CMA) policy on physicians and the pharmaceutical industry (updated in 1998) states that physicians should not engage in "peer selling." A long footnote adds "Peer selling occurs when a pharmaceutical manufacturer directly sponsors a seminar or similar event that focuses on its own products and is designed to enhance the sale of those products. The manufacturer directly engages a physician to conduct the session. This form of participation may be seen as being in contravention of the CMA's Code of Ethics, which prohibits an endorsement of a specific product. Peer selling, as understood in this sense, differs from the sort of situation in which a pharmaceutical manufacturer provides funds to continuing medical education (CME), organizes to sponsor the bona fide educational event on a specific condition, or on specific products. In the latter event the control and structure of the CME event lies in the hands of the CME organizers. Even though the products may be the focus of such a bona fide event, the arm's length nature of the sponsorship by the manufacturer and the fact that the control and structure of the event lie in the hands of the CME organizers, remove it from the realm of advertising and do not constitute an endorsement of the product in question" [23]. It appears that in contradiction of the CMA policy on peer selling, there was a very strong potential influence on physicians from the insurance industry on this occasion.

The Quebec Task Force

The Quebec Task Force [20] was a body organized by an insurance company to examine issues connected with whiplash and to report on them. In this respect it was clear who was paying for the conference and who had determined the matters to be examined by the board. The Task Force was appointed by the Societé de l' Asssurance Automobile du Quebec (SAAQ), a provincial government no-fault insurance carrier located in Canada's second largest province. It comprised clinicians, scientists, and epidemiologists, and conducted an exhaustive review of the scientific literature. It was asked to make public policy recommendations regarding the prevention and treatment of whiplash and associated disorders. The stated reasons for commissioning this study reflected concern with both the magnitude of the problem of whiplash-associated disorders (WADS) and the development of strategies to effectively deal with them. The Quebec Task Force provided a three-part report. The first part described a systematic evaluation of the literature on the treatment of whiplash and concluded, not unreasonably, that few, if any, treatments had adequate evidence to support their use and that the best results appeared to be obtained by undertaking "usual activity" as far as possible after whiplash injury. This is not controversial.

The second major part of the Quebec Task Force Report consisted of a survey of the outcome in a cohort of patients with whiplash claiming benefits from the SAAQ over a period of 1 year. The definition of recovery was based on the decision of the company's adjuster that a claimant was no longer in need of, or entitled to, any continuing benefits. This in itself is a questionable procedure and requires confidence in the balance of judgment and independence of the adjustors. Cessation of benefits and not improvement in pain or return to work defined recovery. This in itself is a questionable procedure and requires confidence in the balance of judgment and the independence of the adjustors. While it is certainly of interest and and importance for insurance companies to know the percentage of individuals whom they expect will not be continuing to receive benefits, the idea that this gives a full measure of recovery is not tenable.

Using this stringent measure the Quebec Task Force reported after evaluating 3014 cases that in 1 year only 1.9% of subjects eligible for inclusion in the study were still not recovered at the end of 12 months. It has to be contrasted with findings from studies from hospital populations in which the percentage of individuals remaining *ill* has been noted to range from 20% to 45% [24]. Gargan and Bannister [24] reported on 50 consecutive patients with soft tissue neck injuries attending an emergency room within 5 days of the accident. After 2 years, 19 (18%) reported they had recovered completely. Radanov and colleagues [25] studied patients referred specifically within the first week after injury by primary care physicians. Twenty-eight (1/7) (24%) were still symptomatic at 12 months. Hildingsson and Toolanen [26] studied 93 consecutive cases referred acutely to an orthopedic department because of a "non-contact injury to the cervical spine resulting from car accidents." At follow-up an average of 2 years after the accident, 43% had discomfort sufficient enough to interfere with their capacity to work. These are regarded as three of the best prospective longitudinal studies. The figure of 1.9% offered by the Quebec Force was widely discordant with these hospital survey figures.

The figures of the Quebec Task Force had a great initial impact in Canada and perhaps in other countries as well in that the authors appeared to have established that if there is anyone still complaining of whiplash after 1 year they could not really blame the particular origin of the illness on the injury received. There is a certain normal incidence of neck pain in the general population and it would have been reasonable with such figures to attribute at least some of that 1.9%, if not all of it, to random events of sickness occurring among the general population. Many people who were involved in rear-end collisions do not suffer from significant whiplash and only about one in seven develop symptoms that lead to a claim for benefits. However among that group of 14% of individuals who have rear-end collisions clearly a much larger percentage than 2% have been found by other investigators to have significant symptoms.

There is a problem with the Quebec Task Force figures [20]. In the middle of the report of the Quebec Task Force we noted the following line saying that "recurrences" "...defined as the recurrence of symptoms of collision-related injuries were found to have occurred in 204 or 6.8% of the study subjects." Remarkably, these subjects were excluded at that point from the study. Taking such a step at this point is curious since recovery was never defined on the basis of symptoms.

In addition to the 6.8% so coyly disclosed, the study's authors had omitted all cases of whiplash in which there were other injuries, amounting to a further 1.1% of cases. When all these are added together the apparent rate of whiplash injury not recovered at 1 year in accordance with the views of the company's own adjuster, is 9.5%, still much lower than the figures found by independent workers, but at least not totally out of line with normal clinical experience.

The cohort study conducted by the Quebec Task Force seems to have been aimed at results that were very insurance-friendly, but rather inimical to the interests of patients. Nevertheless, it was understood from the beginning that this was openly and frankly an insurance company–funded study organized by officials with the company and pursued with some modest help from another interested company (Saskatchewan Government Insurance).

Saskatchewan Government Insurance

The other contribution on the topic of whiplash and its prognosis that attracted much attention was published by Cassidy and colleagues in 2000 [27], based on figures from Saskatchewan Government Insurance (SGI). This study provides a prospective comparison between claimants treated under a tort regime and claimants treated under a no-fault regime. Under the tort regime, while some no-fault benefits were available, individuals also had the right in certain circumstances to sue the tortfeasor (the motorist who is alleged to have caused the damage). SGI is a monopoly provincial government insurer, as is the SAAQ, and the government of Saskatchewan passed a law moving to a totally no-fault system that precludes paying tort damages for pain and suffering with effect from 1 January 1995. Before the new law took effect SGI funded the University of Saskatchewan to commence a survey of an inception cohort with traffic injuries in Saskatchewan comparing 3046 individuals injured under the tort system with 4416 under the subsequent no-fault system. These were refined down from a larger total. Analysis of the data led to the widely cited statement that claimants recover faster if compensation for pain and suffering is not available, as under the no-fault system. As before the criterion for improvement was primarily claim closure, which occurred after 433 days with tort compared with 198 days under no-fault. Cassidy and colleagues [27] also claimed that "The intensity of neck pain, the level of physical function and the presence or absence of depressive symptoms were strongly associated with time to claim closure in both systems." They added, "The elimination of compensation for pain and suffering is associated with a deceased incidence and improved prognosis of whiplash injury."

At this point it might appear that the Saskatchewan study had rehabilitated Henry Miller's usually discredited assertions, notwithstanding their demolition in 1982 by Mendelson.

It is not difficult to believe that when an insurance company has the principal role to play in closing a claim without much opportunity for the claimant to object effectively it may well do so in half the time that would otherwise be required for a case to be heard at law. It is remarkable however that such a conclusion was presented as evidence of medical improvement.

In fact, the data were managed in a way that rather resembles that of the Quebec Task Force. According to the authors "re-openings" were excluded from the analysis. What were "re-openings"? As before with the Quebec Task Force, it seems most likely that many "re-openings" were attributable to patients coming back and complaining that they had been cut-off but that their symptoms had returned when their medication was reduced (perhaps after drug payment benefits were stopped), or they increased their activities by returning to work and found it untenable, or when they even reduced their drugs themselves to see how they would get along. The re-openings discarded from the data set amounted to 2064 or 27%. Cassidy and colleagues [27] originally stated that their reason for dropping these claims was that if SGI closed a claim and it was then re-opened, the re-opened claim "overwrote" the date of the original claim closure and therefore the cases were dropped from review. On being challenged, Cassidy and colleagues [28] stated that they would require ethics approval to return to the documents in question.

This logic raised a red flag and in the light of the Quebec Task Force report promoted a sense of déjà vu. Concern did not abate when a retired adjuster wrote that if a claim was closed and then re-opened she could find it on her computer. It had become easier to obtain such information that was also to be found on the hard copy [29]. In the course of the study, an epidemiologist, who had been appointed to work on the data, resigned on the grounds that she had been pressured to present data in ways that she considered not to be in accordance with proper epidemiological methods.

The original principal investigator, a well-respected professor of orthopedic surgery, also thought that there was cause for concern. He was subsequently dismissed from the study at the request of the funding agency, the insurance company [30]. It is of note that he had objected to the too-close association of an employee of the insurance company with the research team [31].

Many reflections may occur with respect to this story that can be pursued through the references cited. It seems reasonable to conclude that the insurance company had a major influence, not just on the research but also on how the results were presented.

Summary

Evidence acquired through research is increasingly being used to manage medical problems, and, where applicable, to decide on which medically related conditions warrant compensation for disability. Consensus-based guidelines are supposedly prepared by learned individuals, making use of the best evidence and their experiences to provide group wisdom for practicing clinicians. Because bias is always a problem, research strives to minimize bias through scrupulous methodology, while consensus panels work carefully through the constitution of the group and disclosure of conflicts of interest by participants.

Where research is not funded at arm's length by the external funding agency the potential for bias is enormous, especially when substantial funds are at stake, depending on the outcome of the study. In order that future research and consensus group recommendations may result in better care and a fairer compensation system, substantial efforts to minimize bias will be required.

References

[1] Merskey H, Bogduk N. Classification of chronic pain: descriptions of chronic pain syndromes and definitions of pain terms. 2nd edition. Monograph for the Sub-Committee on Taxonomy. International Association for the Study of Pain. Seattle (WA): IASP Press; 1994.

[2] Treede R-D. Pain and hyperalgesia: definitions and theories. In: Cervero F, Jensen TS, editors. Handbook of clinical neurology. Edinburgh, UK: Elsevier; 2006. p. 1–10.

[3] Merskey H, Spear FG. Pain: psychological and psychiatric aspects. London: Bailliere, Tindall & Cassell; 1967.

[4] Inman T. On so-called hysterical pain. BMJ 1858;2:24–5.

[5] Loeser JD. Pain as a disease. In: Cervero F, Jensen TS, editors. Handbook of clinical neurology. Edinburgh, UK: Elsevier; 2006. p. 11–20, 14–15.

[6] Burney F. A mastectomy (1812). In: Hemlow J, editor. Selected letters and journals. Oxford: Clarendon Press; 1986. p. 127–42.

[7] Petit MA. Discours sur la douleur. Delivered at the opening of the Course in Anatomy and Surgery for the General Hospital of Lyons, 19 November 1799. Lyons: Reymann & Co., 1799.

[8] Shorter E. Bedside manners. New York: Simon and Schuster; 1985.

[9] Berridge V. Opiate use and drug control policy in 19th and early 20th century England. London: Free Association Books; 1999.

[10] Merskey H. Post-traumatic stress disorder and shell shock. In: Berrios GE, Porter R, editors. A history of clinical psychiatry. London: Athlone Press; 1995. p. 490–500.

[11] Merskey H. Aspects of hysteria since 1922. In: Freeman HL, Berrios GE, editors. 150 years of British psychiatry. Vol. 2: the aftermath. London: Athlone Press; 1996. p. 5, 89–118.

[12] Schmiedebach HP. Post-traumatic neurosis in nineteenth century Germany: a disease in political, juridical and professional context. Hist Psychiatry 1999;10(37):27–57.

[13] Fordyce WE. Report of the Task Force on Back Pain in the Workplace. International Association for the Study of Pain. Seattle (WA): IASP Press; 1996.

[14] Miller HG. Accident neurosis. BMJ 1961;i:919–25, 992–8.

[15] Mendelson G. Not "cured by a verdict." Effect of legal settlement of compensation claimants. Med J Aust 1982;ii:219–30.

[16] Merskey H, Teasell RW. The disparagement of pain: social influences on medical thinking. Pain Res Manage 2000;5(4):259–70.

[17] Report of the Joint Working Party of the Royal College of Surgeons of England and the College of Anaesthetists. London: Royal College of Surgeons of England; 1990.

[18] Middleton C. Barriers to the provision of effective pain management. Nurs Times 2004; 100(3):42–5.

[19] Canadian Medical Association. Policy summary: physicians and the pharmaceutical industry (Update, 1994). Can Med Assoc J 1994;150:256A–C.

[20] Wolfe F, Allen M, Bennett RM, et al. The fibromyalgia syndrome. A consensus report on fibromyalgia and disability. J Rheumatol 1996;23:534–9.

[21] Yunus MB, Bennett RM, Romano TJ, et al. Fibromyalgia Consensus Report: additional comments. J Clin. Rheumatol 1997;3:324–7.

[22] Merskey H, Teasell RW. The Quebec Task Force on Whiplash-Associated Disorders. Pain Res Manage 1999;4:162–3.

[23] Policy Summary CMA. Physicians and the pharmaceutical industry (update 1994). Can Med Assoc J 1994;150:256A–C.

[24] Gargan MF, Bannister GC. The rate of recovery following whiplash injury. Eur Spine J 1994;3:162–4.

[25] Radanov BP, Sturzenegger M, DeStefano G, et al. Relationship between early somatic radiological and psychosocial findings and outcome during a one-year follow-up in 117 patients with a diagnosis of whiplash who were referred specifically by primary care physicians. Br J Rheumatol 1994;33:442–8.

[26] Hildingsson C, Toolanen G. Outcome after soft tissue injury of the cervical spine. Acta Orthop Scand 1990;6(14):357–9.

[27] Cassidy JD, Carroll LJ, Côté P, et al. Effect of eliminating compensation for pain and suffering on the outcome of insurance claims for whiplash injury. New Engl J Med 2000; 342(16):1179–86.

[28] Cassidy JD, Carroll LJ, Côté P. Effect of eliminating compensation for pain and suffering on the outcome of insurance claims for whiplash injury. N Engl J Med 2000;343:1120.

[29] Kivol K. Saskatchewan government insurance study. Pain Res Manage 2000;5:129–30.

[30] Terry L. Insurance research and medical ethics. Pain Res Manage 2002;7(2):101–6.

[31] Yong-Hing K. Letter to Mr. Colin Clackson: Trial Lawyers Association of Saskatchewan, 3 November 1996.

THE MEDICAL
CLINICS
OF NORTH AMERICA

Med Clin N Am 91 (2007) 45–55

Behavioral Medicine Approaches to Pain

Akiko Okifuji, PhD[a],*, Stacy Ackerlind, PhD[b]

[a]Pain Research and Management Center, Department of Anesthesiology, University of Utah,
615 Arapeen Drive, Suite 200, Salt Lake City, UT 84108, USA
[b]Student Affairs, University of Utah, A Ray Olpin Union Building,
200 S. Central Campus Drive, Room 270, Salt Lake City, UT 84132, USA

In the early 1970s, the term "behavioral medicine" began appearing in the literature as a branch of behavioral science that applies scientific knowledge and techniques to prevention, diagnosis, treatment, and rehabilitation of physical illness and maintenance of physical health [1]. A fundamental aspect of behavioral medicine is the recognition that psychological and behavioral factors reciprocally and dynamically interact with physical health/illness. Linear causality does not exist in this reciprocal relationship. Instead, behavioral medicine interventions assume that by addressing psychosocial and behavioral factors relevant to the illness in question, the overall clinical picture of the condition will improve.

In the early days of pain medicine, treatments for pain patients were primarily biomedical in nature, targeting specific anatomy, physiology, and neurochemistry to alter nociceptive input. However, the proliferation of behavioral research indicates that a number of behavioral and psychological factors contribute to the experience of pain, particularly chronic cases, which has prompted the application of behavioral medicine approaches to pain treatment.

Complex pain cases, particularly noncancer chronic pain, often require multidimensional conceptualization and treatment. Accordingly, multimodal approaches aimed at reduction of pain and resumption of a productive life are considered critical. Behavioral medicine is generally imbedded in a comprehensive multimodal pain treatment program. One of the most commonly used behavioral medicine approaches for pain is cognitive-behavioral therapy, specifically addressing pain-related cognitions and behaviors. Accumulated research in the past 3 decades strongly suggests that

This work was supported by Grant No. AR48888 from the National Institutes of Arthritis, Musculoskeletal, and Skin Diseases to the first author.
* Corresponding author.
E-mail address: akiko.okifuji@hsc.utah.edu (A. Okifuji).

multimodal interventions that include cognitive-behavioral therapy modalities is beneficial and cost-effective [2,3].

Underlying the cognitive-behavioral perspective is the integration of cognitive, affective, and behavioral factors into an overall clinical picture and treatment of pain patients. In the model, each patient is considered as an active processor of external cues that modulates his/her internal state. Psychological variables such as anticipation, avoidance, contingencies of reinforcement, and mood factors are of particular interest. Clearly, the cognitive-behavioral model is not just patients' responses to actual events, but also learned responses to predict and summon appropriate reactions to actual or anticipated events. The cognitive-behavioral framework assumes that how patients perceive their situation and what they expect from their conditions are significant contributors to their health status and disability.

There are five central assumptions that characterize the cognitive-behavioral perspective on pain management (see Box 1). The first assumption is that all people are active processors of information rather than passive entities reacting to events or physical cues. Information is processed through use of well-developed cognitive schemes that people have developed as a result of their learning histories. The process is generally overlearned and automated, and thus people are often not aware that they are operating from a set of assumptions that guide their behavior. Nevertheless, people are constantly engaged in this process in their attempt to make sense of the world around them. People can and do adjust their cognitive schemes to adapt to changing environmental demands.

A second assumption of the cognitive-behavioral perspective is that one's cognitive attributions, beliefs, and expectancies can elicit or modulate affect

---

Box 1. Basic assumptions of cognitive-behavioral treatment

1. People are active processors of information rather than passive reactors to environmental contingencies.
2. Thoughts (for example, appraisals, attributions, expectancies) can elicit or modulate physiological and affective responses, both of which may serve as impetuses for behavior. Conversely, affect, physiology, and behavior can instigate or influence one's thinking processes.
3. Behavior is reciprocally determined by both the environment and the individual.
4. In the same way as people are instrumental in the development and maintenance of maladaptive thoughts, feelings, and behaviors, they can, are, and should be considered active agents of change of their maladaptive modes of responding.

and physiological arousal, both of which may serve as impetuses for behavior. Conversely, affect, physiology, and behavior can instigate or influence one's thinking processes. This cycle is dynamic and continuous, and a causal direction is less of a concern than awareness that this interactive process extends over time with the interaction of thoughts, feelings, physiological activity, and behavior.

The third assumption of the cognitive-behavioral perspective is that behaviors occur as a function of reciprocal interaction between the environment and the individual. Given an event, people respond to the environment, which may in turn alter the environment and elicit others to behave in certain ways. In a very real sense, people are the most prominent contributors to their environments. The chain of such interactions over time makes each person's behavioral pattern unique and idiosyncratic. Ironically, most people are not aware of this process and make external attributions for their failures and successes. For pain patients, it is important to help them recognize how they influence their environment to increase support and decrease hindrances to treatment success.

The final assumption of the cognitive-behavioral perspective is that people create their own reality. Just as they are instrumental in the development and maintenance of maladaptive thoughts, feelings, and behaviors, they can, are, and should be considered active agents of change. Pain patients can replace maladaptive modes of responding with more adaptive ones. Pain patients, no matter how severe their pain and despite their common beliefs to the contrary, are not helpless pawns of fate. They can and should become instrumental in learning and carrying out more effective modes of responding to their environment and their situation.

Behavioral medicine assessment of pain patients

The main vehicle of behavioral medicine assessment is a clinical interview with a patient and, if available and feasible, his or her family members. As supplemental informational sources, standardized self-report inventories may be used. The main goals of assessment are to (1) evaluate psychosocial and behavioral factors relevant to the patient's pain and (2) organize and evaluate the relevant information to direct treatment plans. Attention is also given to identification of any factors that might be impediments to rehabilitation as well as factors that may facilitate the rehabilitative processes.

Typically, the assessment protocol consists of three parts. The first part focuses on understanding a clinical picture of the patient's experience of pain. Specifically, a brief history of pain, learning current pain parameters (eg, quality of pain, time parameters, aggravating/relieving factors), other relevant medical history, and assessing current functional levels, including sleep quality and functional impairment due to pain. It is also important to assess how the patient conceptualizes his or her own pain, the patient's understanding of the potential etiological factors, whether he or she believes adequate diagnostic work has been done, and his or her expectations as to what types of treatments may affect adherence to the treatment regimen and ultimately the success of treatment.

The second part of assessment focuses on gaining a broader understanding of the patient. This includes psychosocial history, including family and personal history of pain, functional abilities and limitations, psychological disorders, and problems with substances (including prescription drugs). This information should help the assessor gain a better understanding of how the patient has historically coped with illness and stress, current life circumstances that may aid/impede treatment efforts, and the level of coping resources available to the patient.

The third part of the assessment is a psychological examination to assess the patient's current mental status, mood functions, and any maladaptive behavioral patterns that may influence the course of pain rehabilitation. Because of the high rate of depression and anxiety among pain patients, it is important to address these issues. All of this information is integrated with biomedical information and is used in treatment planning. There should be a close relationship between the data acquired during the assessment phase and the nature, focus, and goals of the therapeutic regimen.

Cognitive-behavioral therapy: self-management of pain

As noted previously, cognitive-behavioral therapy (CBT) is the most commonly used approach in behavioral medicine for pain patients. There are three main components of CBT for pain: patient education, behavioral skill training, and cognitive-skill training.

Patient education

Since the patient's active participation is critical for successful CBT, it is often essential that patients attain some understanding of the basic psychophysiological processes related to pain, sleep, function, and mood. The difference between acute pain and chronic pain, hurt versus harm concept, and what to expect from rehabilitation processes versus acute pain therapy can set the stage for skill training. Knowledge related to the behavioral principles, such as conditioning, reinforcement, pain/illness behaviors, and how those principles interact with pain and disability can also help patients prepare for the behavioral skills training phase.

Behavioral skills training

Relaxation and controlled breathing exercises are especially useful in the skills-acquisition phase because they can be readily learned by almost all patients. Relaxation and controlled breathing involve behavioral manipulation of the autonomic nervous system by systematically tensing and relaxing various muscle groups, both general and specific to the particular area of pain

reported by patients. These skills are useful to reduce anxiety and stress responses associated with pain and improve sleep. It is important that patients
understand that relaxation is an active process. Many people mistakenly believe that relaxation is a passive process where one rests and avoids working
(eg, laying down in a couch and watching TV). Physiological effects of such
active relaxation can be easily measured with a fingertip thermometer that
tends to indicate a slight increase in finger temperature due to increased
blood flow in the periphery during and after active relaxation [4,5]. Furthermore, it provides a simple demonstration to patients that their behaviors can
alter their physiological states, and thereby substantiate the credibility of behavioral medicine approaches.

Another behavioral skill that is often used in CBT is attentional training.
Attention plays a major role in any perceptual process. The pain experience
tends to be exacerbated by increased attention to pain-related somatic signals
[6]. Because our attentional resources are limited, by actively directing a patient's attention to nonpain stimuli, the available attentional resources
directed toward pain should decrease. This can be achieved by having patients
directly engage in overt behaviors (eg, breathing exercises, progressive muscle
relaxation) or use mental imageries to situations that are typically ones unrelated to pain. Although imagery-based strategies (eg, refocusing attention on
pleasant pain-incompatible scenes) have received much attention, the results
have *not* consistently demonstrated that imagery strategies are uniformly
effective for all patients [7]. The important component as to whether this intervention is effective seems to be the patient's imaginative ability, involvement,
and degree of absorption in using specific images. Guided imagery training is
given to patients to enhance their abilities to use all sensory modalities. The
specifics of the images seem less important than the details of sensory modalities incorporated and the patient's involvement in these images. Patients also
vary in their ability to use distraction techniques as well as what they find to be
an adequate distraction target. The collaborative working relationship
between a therapist and patient becomes essential during this part of training.

A variety of other behavioral skills training can be incorporated into the
treatment plan to meet patients' clinical needs. For example, some patients
experience interpersonal stress to be a major aggravating factor for their
pain. Interpersonal relationships are a key component of an individual's environment. Basic interpersonal skills training in the areas of communication,
assertiveness, and problem-solving skills may help patients better regulate
their stress levels and increase their ability to actively manage their pain.

Cognitive skills training

Typical cognitive training for pain management begins with helping patients understand their own cognitive response system. Specifically, patients
can learn to monitor situational factors that tend to trigger their pain/stress
and what they actually experience emotionally, behaviorally, and physically

when they have pain/stress (see Table 1). In the middle column, patients monitor and understand their own processes that may mediate the relationship between situational factors and the consequential experience. There are a number of potential processes that can be discussed; however, the focus is on cognitive processes that patients learn to monitor and regulate.

Effective self-regulation of pain depends on the individual's specific ways of dealing with pain, adjusting to pain, and reducing or minimizing pain and distress caused by pain through use of coping strategies. Coping strategies include positive self-talk focused on the intention to manage pain and the belief that one is able to execute necessary acts to do so effectively. Through the use of coping strategies, a person has an improved chance of successfully engaging in everyday activities, thereby reducing functional limitations and enhancing his or her sense of control over pain and associated symptoms. It is, however, important to note that effective coping largely depends on various personal (eg, self-efficacy beliefs), situational (eg, work, living arrangements), and psychosocial factors (eg, family history of pain, level of support). Interaction between coping strategies and personal and situational factors may be a critical factor in how coping strategies are implemented. Clinicians need to understand how patients interpret their world through the use of their cognitive systems (eg, self-talk, self-efficacy beliefs, instrumentality).

In cognitive skills training, self-efficacy beliefs are particularly important in treatment. Self-efficacy is defined as a personal conviction that one can effectively handle a situation by executing a course of action to produce a desired outcome [8]. The self-efficacy expectation is a critical mediator of therapeutic change for chronic pain patients [9]. Pain patients' self-efficacy beliefs are largely influenced by their own past success/failure at performing tasks to manage their pain; thus, it is imperative that a therapeutic process leads to an experience of effective performance. Such experience may be created by encouraging patients to undertake a relatively easy task in the beginning and gradually increasing the difficulty to match the difficulty of the desired behavioral repertoire. This developmental process allows self-efficacy to increase. In short, effective coping behaviors are essentially directed by the individual's beliefs that situation demands do not exceed their coping resources.

Another important aspect in cognitive training is to understand specific patients' cognitive repertoires. Tendency to appraise situations negatively is known to deter treatment success [10,11]. Some of the common negative

Table 1
Cognitive behavioral framework for stress/pain management

Stressors	Processes	Stress response
What triggers stress/pain cycle	Modulating processes mediating between stressors and stress responses	What experientially happens to a person in response to stressors • Physiological • Behavioral • Emotional

cognitions are listed in Box 2. In cognitive training, therapists help patients become aware of their own tendency for negative cognitions, and then to exercise the application of alternative ways of appraising the situations. A large number of self-help books and therapy manuals are available to help patients and clinicians go through the process in a step-by-step manner (eg, [12–14]).

Behavioral approach to improve compliance and motivation

One of the critical requirements for successful rehabilitation of chronic pain is that patients adopt an active, participatory role in their treatments. Literature repeatedly indicates that multidisciplinary pain care that includes an activating therapy to restore functioning is effective [2], requiring patients to modify lifestyles to incorporate various physical activities. Such adaptation is often difficult even for healthy individuals; a report to the surgeon general [15] shows that 50% of those who sign up with gyms at the beginning of a year drop out within 6 months. Thus, it is not surprising that pain patients find it difficult to comply with regular physical activity regimens, even with the implementation of CBT to improve coping.

Therapeutic effort to help patients comply with their treatment regimen is of a growing interest. Long-term treatment success depends on regular adherence to recommended self-care regimens for people suffering from chronic pain conditions [16]. Historically, clinicians invest less energy in patients who show little commitment to therapies. However, as we increasingly

---

Box 2. Examples of common negative cognitive patterns

Polarizing pattern: Black-and-white thinking. If a patient's performance falls short of perfect, the patient sees himself or herself as a total failure, leading to high expectation that is often unattainable.

Overgeneralization pattern: A patient generalizes beyond the specific facts of a situation, and sees a single negative experience as a never-ending pattern of defeat.

Catastrophizing pattern: A patient consistently assumes the worst possible outcomes. The patient's understanding of his or her own plight is extremely negative and the patient tends to interpret relatively minor problems as major catastrophes.

Filtering pattern: A patient focuses on a single negative detail, rather than a whole picture, of the event and lets the single detail characterize the entire experience.

Emotional reasoning pattern: A patient assumes that his or her negative emotions reflect the reality. "I really feel it, therefore this must be true."

face issues related to chronic illness that are closely tied with people's lifestyle issues, helping patients comply with functional regimens has become a critical clinical issue in pain management.

Motivation Enhancement Therapy

Motivation Enhancement Therapy (MET), developed by William Miller and his colleagues [17], is one of the therapeutic methods that targets patient motivation. MET is based on the assumption that people vary in their degree of readiness for change. Stated differently, patients are considered to be in a certain motivational stage of change. MET strategies are organized to help a patient move from a low level of motivation (or a lower level in the model) to increased motivation (or a higher level in the model) via therapist-patient interactions. Each of the motivational stages is presented in Box 3.

MET is a problem-focused, therapist-directed approach aiming to help patients enhance their commitment and motivation for treatment. MET offers a collection of therapeutic techniques to help patients (1) clearly recognize their problems, (2) perform a personal cost-benefit analysis of their therapeutic or countertherapeutic behaviors, (3) develop consistency between their therapy goals and motivation, and (4) internalize motivational thoughts via improved self-efficacy.

MET has been tested for facilitating change to reduce problem behaviors, such as smoking [18,19], problem drinking [20,21], problem gambling [22], eating disorders [23] and high risk sexual behaviors [24,25]. MET has also been shown to increase healthy behaviors such as promoting exercise with myocardial infarction patients [26], adherence to glucose control regimen in patients with diabetes [27], and mammography screening [28].

Motivation Enhancement Therapy for pain patients

MET is based on the assumption that people vary in their levels of commitment and motivation for complying with activating regimens. There are

---

Box 3. Stages of change

1. **Precontemplative stage:** Patient does not perceive a need to change and actively resists change.
2. **Contemplation stage:** Patient begins to see a need for change and may consider making a change in the future
3. **Preparation stage:** Patient feels ready to change and takes a first concrete (behavioral) change
4. **Action stage:** Patient actively engages in behaviors consistent with regimen
5. **Maintenance stage:** Patient executes plans to sustain the changes made

several key components in MET [29] that facilitate increased motivation to change maladaptive behavioral patterns and replace them with more adaptive ones. First, a clinician should refrain from judgmental attitudes and responses. Empathy and reflection of patients' feelings is useful at the early stage of MET. Rolling with resistance (ie, not pressuring the patient to change) is another essential interpersonal strategy used in MET. The clinician and patient should remain on the same side, thereby not increasing resistance to change. One of the easy pitfalls is for a clinician to push his or her agenda and as a consequence, let the patient present a counter-argument for why he or she should not engage in therapeutic effort. By going with the patient's resistance, the clinician facilitates the formation of a therapeutic alliance, which is critical to increase the patient's motivation to change. Second, the clinician helps patients to identify specific discrepancies between what they want from pain care (eg, "I want to get well and go out more often") and what they actually do (eg, "I can't do my exercise because I have no time and I don't feel well"). By focusing on the discrepancy, patients gain insight that their maladaptive behaviors and attitudes are actually preventing them from obtaining their goal of getting better. This insight promotes the patient's motivation to change. Similarly, patients benefit greatly from engaging in "decisional balance analysis" of their own behaviors. For example, patients list their "pros" for exercising, as well as for not exercising, and "cons" for exercising as well as for not exercising, which can be discussed and used to increase the discrepancy between the patient's goals and actions. The decisional balance analysis helps patients gain a better understanding of their behavior, in this case, why they do not want to exercise. Through this process, patients become more aware of their role in maintaining maladaptive behaviors as well as identifying strategies to engage in more adaptive behaviors.

Another essential feature of MET is to provide a supportive environment to nurture a sense of self-efficacy and ultimately a patient's ability to change his or her behaviors. By understanding that change is a process that the patient has control over, patients realize that change is possible. With increased self-efficacy beliefs comes a sense of responsibility and an awareness that it is patients themselves who will choose to engage in therapeutic efforts and execute them. MET is a clinician-directed approach that is heavily patient-centered. Detailed descriptions of the specific MET approach are beyond the scope of this paper. Interested readers may find a comprehensive book by Miller and Rollnick helpful [29].

Summary

Managing pain patients can be a challenging task for many clinicians because of the complexity of the condition. Pain by definition [30] is a multifactorial phenomenon for which biomedical factors interact with a web of psychosocial and behavioral factors. Behavioral medicine approaches for pain generally address specific cognitive and behavioral factors relevant to pain, thereby aiming to modify the overall pain experience and help restore functioning and quality of life in pain patients.

Behavioral medicine focuses on patients' motivation to comply with a rehabilitative regimen, particularly those with chronic, disabling pain. Since patients' own commitment and active participation in a therapeutic program are critical for the successful rehabilitation, the role that behavioral medicine can play is significant. It is not unreasonable to state that success outcomes of the rehabilitative approach depend on how effectively behavioral medicine can be integrated into the overall treatment plan. Past research in general supports this assertion, demonstrating clinical benefit and cost-effectiveness of multidisciplinary interventions that include behavioral medicine. Some of the approaches listed in this paper can be incorporated into clinicians' practice regardless of specialties, and such practice will likely provide helpful venues for managing pain patients.

References

[1] Gentry WD. Behavioral medicine: A new research paradigm. In: Gentry WD, editor. Handbook of behavioral medicine. New York: Guilford; 1984.
[2] Okifuji A. Interdisciplinary pain management with pain patients: evidence for its effectiveness. Sem Pain Med 2003;1(2):110–9.
[3] Turk DC. Clinical effectiveness and cost-effectiveness of treatments for patients with chronic pain. Clin J Pain 2002;18(6):355–65.
[4] Bacon M, Poppen R. A behavioral analysis of diaphragmatic breathing and its effects on peripheral temperature. J Behav Ther Exp Psychiatry 1985;16(1):15–21.
[5] Jacobson AM, Manschreck TC, Silverberg E. Behavioral treatment for Raynaud's disease: a comparative study with long-term follow-up. Am J Psychiatry 1979;136(6):844–6.
[6] McCabe C, Lewis J, Shenker N, et al. Don't look now! Pain and attention. Clin Med 2005; 5(5):482–6.
[7] Fernandez E, Turk DC. The utility of cognitive coping strategies for altering pain perception: a meta-analysis. Pain 1989;38(2):123–35.
[8] Bandura A. Self-efficacy: toward a unifying theory of behavioral change. Psychol Rev 1977; 84(2):191–215.
[9] Council JR, Ahern DK, Follick MJ, et al. Expectancies and functional impairment in chronic low back pain. Pain 1988;33(3):323–31.
[10] Cook AJ, Degood DE. The cognitive risk profile for pain: development of a self-report inventory for identifying beliefs and attitudes that interfere with pain management. Clin J Pain 2006;22(4):332–45.
[11] Tota-Faucette ME, Gil KM, Williams DA, et al. Predictors of response to pain management treatment. The role of family environment and changes in cognitive processes. Clin J Pain 1993;9(2):115–23.
[12] Caudill-Slosberg M. Managing pain before it manages you. Revised edition. New York: Guilford Press; 2001.
[13] Thorn B. Cognitive therapy for chronic pain: a step-by-step guide. New York: Guilford Press; 2004.
[14] Turk DC, Winter F. The pain survival guide: how to reclaim your life. Washington, DC: American Psychological Association; 2005.

[15] US Department of Health and Human Services. Physical activity and health: a report of the Surgeon General. Atlanta (GA): Centers for Disease Control and Prevention, National Center for Chronic Disease Prevention; 1996.

[16] Turk DC, Rudy TE. Neglected topics in the treatment of chronic pain patients—relapse, noncompliance, and adherence enhancement. Pain 1991;44(1):5–28.

[17] Miller W. Motivational interviewing with problem drinkers. Behav Psychother 1983;11: 147–72.

[18] Town GI, Fraser P, Graham S, et al. Establishment of a smoking cessation programme in primary and secondary care in Canterbury. N Z Med J 2000;113(1107):117–9.

[19] Velasquez MM, Hecht J, Quinn VP, et al. Application of motivational interviewing to pre-natal smoking cessation: training and implementation issues. Tob Control 2000;9(Suppl 3): III36–40.

[20] Brown RL, Saunders LA, Bobula JA, et al. Remission of alcohol disorders in primary care patients. Does diagnosis matter? J Fam Pract 2000;49(6):522–8.

[21] Handmaker NS, Miller WR, Manicke M. Findings of a pilot study of motivational inter-viewing with pregnant drinkers. J Stud Alcohol 1999;60(2):285–7.

[22] Hodgins DC, Currie SR, el-Guebaly N. Motivational enhancement and self-help treatments for problem gambling. J Consult Clin Psychol 2001;69(1):50–7.

[23] Feld R, Woodside DB, Kaplan AS, et al. Pretreatment motivational enhancement therapy for eating disorders: a pilot study. Int J Eat Disord 2001;29(4):393–400.

[24] Carey MP, Braaten LS, Maisto SA, et al. Using information, motivational enhancement, and skills training to reduce the risk of HIV infection for low-income urban women: a second randomized clinical trial. Health Psychol 2000;19(1):3–11.

[25] Kalichman SC, Cherry C, Browne-Sperling F. Effectiveness of a video-based motivational skills-building HIV risk- reduction intervention for inner-city African American men. J Con-sult Clin Psychol 1999;67(6):959–66.

[26] Song R, Lee H. Managing health habits for myocardial infarction (MI) patients. Int J Nurs Stud 2001;38(4):375–80.

[27] Smith DE, Heckemeyer CM, Kratt PP, et al. Motivational interviewing to improve adher-ence to a behavioral weight-control program for older obese women with NIDDM. A pilot study. Diabetes Care 1997;20(1):52–4.

[28] Bernstein J, Mutschler P, Bernstein E. Keeping mammography referral appointments: motivation, health beliefs, and access barriers experienced by older minority women. J Mid-wifery Womens Health 2000;45(4):308–13.

[29] Miller W, Rollnick S. Motivational interviewing: preparing people for change. 2nd edition. New York: Guilford Press; 2002.

[30] International Association for the Study of Pain. Classification of chronic pain. Descriptions of chronic pain syndromes and definitions of pain terms. Pain 1986;3:S217.

ELSEVIER
SAUNDERS

Med Clin N Am 91 (2007) 57–95

THE MEDICAL
CLINICS
OF NORTH AMERICA

Physical Medicine Rehabilitation Approach to Pain

Steven P. Stanos, DO[a,b,*], James McLean, MD[a,c],
Lynn Rader, MD[a,b]

[a]Department of Physical Medicine and Rehabilitation, Northwestern University,
Feinberg School of Medicine, 303 East Chicago Ave., Chicago, IL 60611, USA
[b]Chronic Pain Care Center, Rehabilitation Institute of Chicago, 1030 N. Clark Street,
Suite 320, Chicago, IL 60610, USA
[c]Sports and Spine Rehabilitation Center, Rehabilitation Institute of Chicago,
1030 N. Clark Street, 5th Floor, Chicago, IL 60610, USA

The physiatric model of care is based on a fundamental understanding of the individuals' unique condition as it relates to the concept of (1) impairment, (2) disability, and (3) handicap [1]. Impairment is the psychologic, physical, or functional loss or abnormality. Disability is a restriction or lack of ability to perform activities due to related impairments. Handicap is the disadvantage that an individual possesses due to the impairment or disability that affects the patient's fulfillment of life roles in society (Box 1). A patient-centered approach is necessary to effectively address these important individual concepts. A team-centered approach focuses on helping patients to achieve individual goals, which enables them to improve physical and psychosocial function, decrease pain, and improve quality of life. By working together, the rehabilitation team is able to help patients achieve better outcomes than could be achieved by an individual practitioner. Treatment models include a continuum of care based on patient severity and needs, with increasing complexity of treatment philosophies and need for communication and decreasing individual team-member autonomy [2]. Focused treatment programs for acute conditions may involve individual physical therapy directed by the physiatrist, followed by a coordinated program including ongoing communication with the patient's case manager and therapist. With chronic pain conditions, more diverse assessment and treatment teams include multi- and interdisciplinary programs. In the multidisciplinary model, patient care is planned and managed by a team

---

* Corresponding author.
  E-mail address: sstanos@ric.org (S.P. Stanos).

0025-7125/07/$ - see front matter © 2006 Elsevier Inc. All rights reserved.
doi:10.1016/j.mcna.2006.10.014
medical.theclinics.com

Box 1. World Health Organization definitions of impairment, disability, and handicap

Impairment: "Any loss or abnormality of psychological,
    physiological, or anatomic structure or function"
Disability: "Any restriction or lack (resulting from an impairment)
    of ability to perform an activity in the manner or within the
    range considered normal for a human being"
Handicap: "A disadvantage for a given individual, resulting from
    an impairment or a disability, that limits or prevents the
    fulfillment of a role that is normal (depending on age, sex, and
    social and cultural factors) for that individual"

---

leader. This model is often hierarchical, with one or two individuals direct-ing the services of a range of team members, many with individual goals. Box 2 lists some of the specialists who are commonly part of a comprehen-sive pain rehabilitation team. Treatment may be delivered at different facil-ities or centers. Even more collaborative is the interdisciplinary model, involving team members working together toward a common goal. Team members are able to communicate and consult with other team members on an ongoing basis, facilitated by regular, face-to-face meetings. In this model, team members possess a combination of skills that no single individ-ual demonstrates alone.

This article provides a description of the basic framework of approaching acute and chronic pain conditions with an important focus on the compre-hensive functionally based history and physical examination that includes assessment of gait pattern, posture, strength, and balance. This approach helps to more clearly identify physical impairments and, in turn, lead to a more appropriate treatment plan. In addition, this article reviews

---

Box 2. Members of a pain rehabilitation team

Physiatrists
Rehabilitation nurses
Physical therapists
Occupational therapists
Recreation therapists
Speech language pathologists
Psychologists
Nutritionists
Social workers
Vocational rehabilitation counselors

individual team roles and treatment responsibilities. Various assessment techniques and treatment strategies are discussed. Finally, the application of the continuum of care is applied to acute and chronic pain conditions commonly encountered, including low back pain–related disorders, myofascial pain, and fibromyalgia (FM).

Management continuum for acute and chronic pain

In acute pain syndromes, the experience of pain is often directly linked to an underlying tissue injury. For example, an acute episode of low back pain may be due to a herniated fifth lumbar (L5) disc. Receptors in the outer annulus fibrosus of the disc and surrounding neural tissue transmit signals to the dorsal horn where the signals are first modulated [3] and then ascend to higher brain levels where the multidimensional experience of pain is perceived [4]. In treating patients who have acute pain syndromes, the three important goals are acute management, rehabilitation, and prevention of further, future injury. The acute pain and inflammation should initially be managed using the traditional acronym RICE: rest, ice, compression, and elevation. Oral medications, bracing, therapy, or injections can be used during the initial time following the injury to help alleviate symptoms and aid in the normal healing process. As symptoms begin to resolve, the next phase should focus on addressing factors that may have predisposed the patient to injury. Finally and most importantly, rehabilitation should be geared toward educating the patient about what they have to do to avoid incurring the same injury or similar injuries in the future.

For the patient who has an acute herniated L5 disc, initial management may include several days of relative rest, ice on the lower back, and possibly oral anti-inflammatory medications. Corticosteroid injections can be used to reduce inflammation in selected patients. Physical therapy focuses on normalizing range of motion (ROM) and emphasizing postures that will unload the herniated disc and facilitate healing. As symptoms resolve, biomechanical deficits that may have led to the disc herniation can be addressed. Some of these may include weakness in the core musculature; hamstring inflexibility; decreased hip ROM, causing increased stress on the lumbar spine; previous injury elsewhere in the kinetic chain, resulting in maladaptive adaptations; or poor lifting biomechanics. At the conclusion of treatment, the patient is given recommendations about exercises and lifestyle modifications to help reduce the likelihood of recurrence of the disc herniation.

Patients who fail to see a complete resolution of pain may continue to experience pain and develop psychologic and social distress. A more comprehensive approach is in order when dealing with patients who have persistent pain. In effectively managing chronic pain, the biomedical model of injury is inadequate due to its focus on biologic determinants of disease and illness while inherently ignoring psychologic and behavioral aspects of pain and pain-related suffering. A biopsychosocial approach, as described by

Engel [5], equally embraces the physiologic, psychologic, and social determinants of illness and serves as the foundation of the multidisciplinary and
interdisciplinary pain continuum [6,7].

The role of the physician

The first role of the physician in the management of patients who have
pain is to establish a complete and accurate diagnostic assessment. Without
a clear diagnosis or an understanding of contributing musculoskeletal
impairments, rehabilitation is not likely to be effective and could possibly
contribute to ongoing pain or re-injury. Arriving at this diagnosis involves
a complete history, a comprehensive physical assessment, and appropriate
use of laboratory and radiologic testing. After a diagnosis is reached, the
physician develops a comprehensive plan of care, prioritizing short- and
long-term goals. Individual treatment plans focus on a wide range of areas
including a rational pharmacotherapy approach (ie, analgesia, improved
mood, and restoring quality sleep); physical or occupational therapy; cognitive and behavioral treatments (ie, counseling and relaxation training);
vocational rehabilitation; and patient education. The physiatric approach
encourages a stepwise approach that starts with exercise and noninvasive
means and progresses to more interventional procedures when necessary as
a means of more aggressively controlling pain and helping the patient progress through active therapies. Finally, re-introduction of previous leisure and
sport activities is pursued with progression guided by the therapist.

A physiatric history

A physiatric pain history starts like any standard evaluation of pain. This
evaluation includes identifying the onset of the pain, precipitating events,
location, character, quality, and relieving and exacerbating factors, with
an additional focus on pain-related functional changes. Previous diagnostic
tests and treatments are reviewed. The analysis of function may vary
dramatically based on individual patient characteristics (ie, age, vocation,
leisure interests, and medical comorbidities). For example, a treatment
plan for a collegiate runner may focus entirely on returning the patient to
a previous level of competitive running, whereas for a 70-year-old woman
who has an acute thoracic compression fracture, her functional goals may
include independently dressing herself and taking care of her home. A functional assessment may be done informally or by using a standardized scale.
The Functional Independence Measure is commonly used by rehabilitation
professionals (Box 3) [8]. Significant variability exists in chronic pain
patients with regard to how one's individual pain condition affects function.
For example, consider a 40-year-old male construction worker who has
severe, progressive low back pain. He reports additional frustration with
his inability to tolerate his normal required physical job demands and fears

---

Box 3. Levels of functional independence by the Functional Independence Measure

Complete dependence
1. Total assistance: subject does <25% with assistance
2. Maximal assistance: subject does 25%–50% with assistance

Modified dependence
3. Moderate assistance: subject does 50%–75% with assistance
4. Minimal assistance: subject does 75%–100% with assistance
5. Supervision: subject does 100% without assistance but needs supervision

Independence
6. Modified independence: independent with assistive devices
7. Complete independence: independent without devices and performs tasks timely and safely

---

Scores are assessed for various activities of daily living including self-care, bowel and bladder management, transfers, ambulation, communication, and social integration.

---

possible job termination. The assessment may include identifying more specific job demands, conditions at the workplace, and job-related stressors and work relationships (ie, patient–employer, coworkers). Another patient, an elderly woman who has progressive left hip osteoarthritic pain, reports having more difficulty caring for herself due to difficulty dressing herself and loss of mobility due to worsening walking tolerance. Her assessment may focus more on difficulty with specific tasks that she encounters on a daily basis. With that information, the physical examination may more specifically examine hip and lumbar ROM, functional mobility, balance, and ability to rise efficiently from a seating position. In turn, treatment may first focus on adaptive equipment for dressing, initiating gait training exercises, and providing the patient the necessary resources for assisting her with community transportation.

Finally and most importantly, the physiatric history assesses for the factors that will serve to motivate the patient to reach their goals. Consider a competitive runner who has an overuse injury. Runners, like many athletes, are often willing to accept a certain amount of pain or injury to continue training. Suggesting relative rest to this patient as a means of helping to limit injury may not be successful; however, emphasizing how a more balanced training regimen can improve the patient's long-term performance may allow for a paradigm shift, leading to a change in behavior and a successful rehabilitation outcome.

Comprehensive physical assessment

Physical examination

A physiatric musculoskeletal examination includes a complete examination of the painful area including bony structures, cartilage, joints, ligaments, tendons, bursa, nerves, and skin. Equally important is a more global evaluation of posture, core strength, balance, and gait. Performing a proficient physical examination is a fundamental part of identifying pain generators, diagnosing and identifying potential areas of dysfunction, narrowing the clinical differential diagnosis, and establishing a rational treatment plan. The following sections describe important aspects of a global musculoskeletal assessment and how the findings of this examination can help guide treatment.

Illness behavior

Although often overlooked or recorded in routine examinations and reports, patient "pain behaviors" ("illness behavior") are important parts of the comprehensive chronic pain assessment. Pain behaviors are based on operant contingency models of reinforcement and act as a means for the patient to communicate to the environment that he or she is experiencing pain or distress [9]. These behavioral manifestations of pain (ie, grimacing, complaining, and inactivity) may be positively reinforced, for example, by obtaining attention from family members and being excused from undesirable obligations such as work or pain-provoking activities. Many times, these reinforcement contingencies remain long after the precipitation injury (ie, tissue trauma) has resolved. Other pain behaviors include guarding, bracing, rubbing the painful area, facial grimacing, and sighing [10,11]. Pain behaviors have been found to correlate with self-report measures of pain intensity, pain disability, and self-efficacy [12] and may serve as targets for cognitive and behavioral treatment and, in turn, be "unlearned."

Waddell and Main [13] described illness behavior as "what people say and do to express and communicate they are ill." They classically described five general categories of nonanatomic signs (tenderness, simulation, distraction, regional complaints, and over-reaction) in patients who have low back pain and have what are commonly referred to as Waddell signs (WS) (Box 4) [11]. In their initial study, Waddell and Main [13] found that patients who displayed at least three signs were more likely to have evidence of psychosocial distress. These signs were not intended to be signs of, or a test for, malingering (the intentional production of false or grossly exaggerated physical or psychologic symptoms). It is unfortunate that WS have been routinely used in this regard in clinical practice, something that should be done with significant caution. Controlled studies have demonstrated no consistent evidence that WS are associated with malingering or secondary gain, which is defined as interpersonal advantages that one obtains as the result of injury or disease [14]. Pain

---

Box 4. Waddell symptoms and signs

Waddell symptoms
1. Pain at the tip of the tailbone
2. Whole leg pain
3. Whole leg numbness
4. Whole leg giving way
5. Complete absence of any spells with very little pain in the last year
6. Intolerance of, or reactions to, many treatments
7. Emergency admission to hospital with simple backache

Waddell signs
1. Tenderness: superficial or nonanatomic
2. Simulation tests: axial loading or simulated rotation
3. Distraction tests: physical examination finding is retested with the patient distracted (ie, straight leg raise, seated and supine)
4. Regional changes: weakness or sensory change
5. Over-reaction: exaggerated response to physical examination

---

behaviors should be described on an individual basis as observed during the physical examination. Of interest, Fishbain and colleagues [15] demonstrated that WS were not associated with physician perception of effort exaggeration and found evidence that WS decreased with comprehensive pain treatment.

Posture

Posture is defined as the position of the body at one point in time and is influenced by each of the joints of the body. Proper posture is achieved when the joints line up in such a way as to create the least amount of stress and muscle activation as possible. Poor or dysfunctional postures promote abnormal stresses on the joints and can lead to tissue trauma and eventually pain. For example, forward flexed lumbar posture has been found to correlate with amount of vertebral pain, muscular impairments, motor function, and disability in elderly women [16]. In standing, normal posture includes cervical and lumbar lordosis and a slight thoracic kyphosis. In addition, the examiner should assess the position of the head in relation to the shoulders and assess more global, side-to-side asymmetries. For example, one may observe a superiorly positioned (elevated) right shoulder and a superior (elevated) left iliac crest due to pelvic obliquity and malalignment. Posture may be observed indirectly during the patient interview or formally during the physical examination. Exaggeration or flattening of the relatively normal cervical, thoracic, and lumbar curves is often seen in chronic spine and soft tissue injury conditions. Pelvic asymmetry has been shown to alter body mechanics in sitting and standing, placing various segments under strain, contributing to musculoskeletal pain [17]. It is important to evaluate the patient in his or her normal sitting position. Poor sitting posture places excess strain on multiple structures including the lumbar discs, cervical discs, and the low back and cervical musculature. Postural training, worksite evaluations, lumbar rolls, core strengthening, and stretching of tight musculature can help to improve poor sitting posture. Fig. 1 shows examples of normal and abnormal sitting postures.

Range of motion and muscle imbalances

ROM, muscle strength, and balance should be assessed because deficits in this area can affect a patient's ability to perform the activities of daily living and achieve efficient functional mobility. Active ROM, active assistive ROM, and passive ROM can be assessed for each joint. The examiner should note general hypermobility or hypomobility, side-to-side differences in ROM, and which of the movements result in pain. The findings on ROM

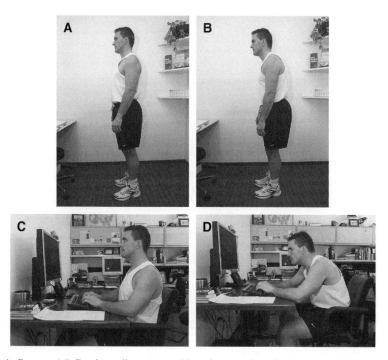

Fig. 1. Posture. (*A*) Good standing posture. Note the normal cervical and lumbar lordosis and thoracic kyphosis. (*B*) Poor standing posture. The shoulders are rounded forward. There is a loss of lumbar lordosis and an exaggeration of the thoracic kyphosis. (*C*) Good sitting posture. The normal cervical, thoracic, and lumbar curvatures are maintained. (*D*) Poor sitting posture. The shoulders are rounded forward. The there is a loss of the normal lumbar and thoracic curvatures. The neck is in compensatory hyperextension.

testing combined with the results of manual muscle testing may lead to objective findings of muscle imbalances about a joint. This concept has been well described by Janda and colleagues [18–20] as the upper-crossed and pelvic-crossed syndromes. An upper-crossed syndrome is characterized by contracted and hypertonic postural muscles (pectoralis major and upper trapezius) and lengthened phasic muscles (rhomboids, serratus anterior, middle and lower trapezius), which may present with related neck and shoulder pain and headaches. Pelvic-crossed syndrome is characterized by contracted hip flexors and lumbar extensors and weak, lengthened phasic muscles (abdominals and gluteus maximus) and may present with chronic low back and buttock pain.

Core strength

The "core" has been likened to a box, with the abdominal muscles in the front, the diaphragm as the roof, and the pelvic floor and hip muscles as the bottom. It includes more than 20 pairs of muscle groups that stabilize spinal structures and the pelvis and coordinate movements during functional tasks such as bending, lifting, and squatting [21]. Efficient functioning of the core helps to distribute, absorb, and limit translational and shearing forces. The outer, more superficial group of muscles is composed of predominantly fast-twitch fibers. These muscles are therefore capable of producing large torque forces, greater speed, and larger arcs of motion (Box 5). The deeper muscles lay closer to the spine and are composed predominantly of slow twitch muscle fibers. These muscles help control segmental motion and help maintain mechanical stiffness of the spine. In one study, operative patients who had unilateral low back pain had evidence of ipsilateral multifidi atrophy (10%–30%) compared with the contralateral side [22]. Weakness of these deep core muscles has been implicated as a precipitator and contributor to the development of chronic low back pain.

Box 5. Core muscles

Superficial core musculature
Rectus abdominus
Erector spinae
External obliques

Deep core musculature
Transverse abdominus
Multifidi
Internal obliques
Deep transversospinalis
Pelvic floor musculature

There are several ways to assess for core strength. A commonly used test is assessing for Trendelenberg's sign during a single-leg stance (Fig. 2). The examiner stands behind the patient and asks him or her to stand on the leg that is being assessed. In an individual who does not have hip weakness, the pelvis remains level. In a patient who has gluteus medius weakness, however, the contralateral hip drops because the ipsilateral hip abductor is not sufficiently strong to stabilize the pelvis. Another test that can be easily performed in the clinic is the "bridge" (Fig. 3). The patient lies supine with his or her knees and hips flexed and feet on the table. The patient then lifts the pelvis while keeping the upper back and feet stabilized on the examination table. The examiner looks for any unsteadiness or pelvic tilting. To make the test more difficult or to assess for more subtle weakness, the patient can additionally be asked to lift one leg off the table and maintain the leg in alignment with the contralateral femur.

Balance and stability

A closely related concept to core strength is balance and stability. Patients who have weak core musculature often demonstrate deficits in this area. These deficits may lead to increased stress in other parts of the body and an increased risk of injury. Tissue injury may then result in more core weakness and instability, resulting in a vicious cycle. In one study, patients who had low back pain demonstrated less balance and postural stability than those who did not have low back pain [23]. In addition, anticipatory postural adjustments, those that precede voluntary movements to stabilize

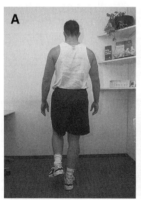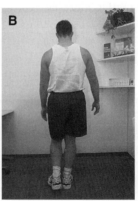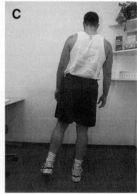

Fig. 2. Trendelenberg's sign. (*A*) Patients who do not have hip gluteus medius weakness are able to maintain the alignment of the hips during a single-leg stance. Note that the iliac crests are at the same level on the left and the right. (*B*) Note the subtle drop of the pelvis on the left. This drop occurs with right gluteus medius weakness and is called the Trendelenberg's sign. (*C*) Patients who have gluteus medius weakness often walk with a compensated Trendelenberg's gait. During stance phase of the affected side, the patient leans the trunk over the stance leg to gain stability and circumducts the contralateral leg.

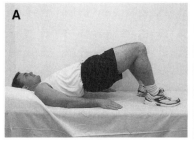
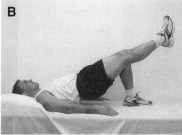
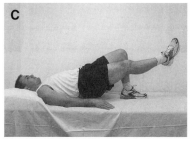

Fig. 3. The "bridge." (*A*) The patient lies supine with knees flexed and feet on the table. The patient elevates the pelvis while maintaining a neutral spine and pelvic alignment. (*B*) To make the exercise more difficult, the patient can alternatively elevate the right and left legs while maintaining the pelvic alignment. (*C*) When core weakness is present, the patient will not be able to maintain the neutral pelvic alignment.

the spine, are abnormally coordinated in patients who have chronic low back pain, primarily due to impaired deep trunk muscle strength [24,25].

Balance can be assessed in various ways. A simple method is to have the patient stand on one leg. A patient who has impaired balance may be unsteady, sway, or be unable to safely lift up one leg without losing balance. If the patient is able perform a single-leg stance without difficulty, then the exercise can be made more challenging by having the patient stand on one leg and perform a single-leg squat. Patients who have poor balance often flail their arms and go into excessive genu valgum (knee angles medial compared with foot) as they "corkscrew" through the ROM (Fig. 4). To detect differences in balance in athletes or well-conditioned individuals, the maneuver may be progressed to a more challenging level by having the patient extend the unsupported leg out into the frontal, sagittal, and transverse planes or by having the patient close his or her eyes.

Gait

Normal gait may be categorized into two phases and seven parameters (Box 6) [26]. Understanding the normal gait cycle helps the examiner identify gait deviations that occur in common pathologic conditions. For example, in a normal individual, stance phase represents 60% of the gait cycle, whereas swing phase represents 40% of the gait cycle. Often, with acute or

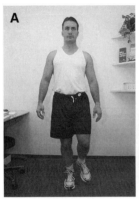
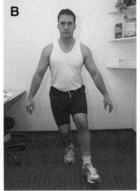
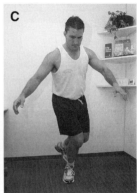

Fig. 4. Single-leg stance and single-leg squat. (*A*) Patients who have good balance will be able to perform the maneuver without falling and with minimal swaying. (*B*) To make the test more difficult, a single-leg squat can be performed. Note that the knee, foot, and hip alignment are maintained. (*C*) Patients who have poor core strength and impaired balance often "corkscrew" as they perform the squat. Notice the pronation, genu valgum, hip rotation, and flailing arms.

chronic pain conditions in the lower extremity, an antalgic gait pattern is seen. On the affected side, less time is spent in stance phase as the patient shifts his or her weight to the contralateral side to avoid pain. This pain-avoidance pattern can cause problems in other areas including the compensated hip, knee, and ankle joint or related soft tissue structures. Another common gait deviation is the compensated Trendelenberg's gait. Consider a patient who has right gluteus medius weakness resulting in a positive Trendelenberg's sign and poor balance when performing a single-leg stance. To maintain the contralateral hip in alignment during stance phase, the patient often leans over the affected hip to compensate for the weak hip abductors. The patient may also circumduct or swing the contralateral leg to prevent dragging the foot (see Fig. 4).

When possible, gait should be assessed when the patient enters the examination room. Subsequently, a more detailed examination of gait can be performed with the formal examination, looking for inconsistencies. For a complete assessment of gait, the patient should be without shoes or socks and wearing minimal clothing, allowing the examiner to assess the shoulders, low back, hips, knees, ankles, and feet. Successive trials should be performed and the examiner should assess each of these joints independently. It is important to remember that gait deviations in one area usually affect other areas of the body. For example, a significant pes planus (flat foot) can affect the forces at the knee and at the hip during gait. A hip flexion contracture results in excessive lumbar lordosis (extension of the lumbar spine relative to the sacrum and pelvis) and can exacerbate painful low back pain conditions such as facet arthropathy due to increased forces and strain through the facet joints caused by relative hyperextension of the lumbar spine as a means of maintaining standing posture.

Box 6. Phases of gait and important gait parameters

Phases of gait
Stance: 60% of the walking cycle; shortened on the painful side
Swing: 40% of the walking cycle; lengthened on the painful side

Important parameters of gait
Width of support: distance between feet; normally 2–4 inches;
  larger when pathology of the dorsal columns or an ataxic gait
  is present
Step length: distance between sequential corresponding points
  of contact by opposite feet; normally 14–16 inches
Step length: shortened on the pain-free side
Stride length: distance between sequential corresponding points
  of contact by the same foot; normally 30 inches
Pelvic and trunk rotation: helps to elongate the leg, increasing
  step length and stride length
Cadence: number of steps per minute; normally 100 steps per
  minute
Center of gravity: 2 inches anterior to the second sacral vertebrae

---

Kinetic chain

After the completion of the musculoskeletal examination, having a firm understanding of the kinetic chain helps the clinician to interpret the patient's deficits and to develop a treatment regimen. The kinetic chain concept is based on the fundamental premise that for functional movement in space, each link of the body must move in a coordinated manner. The sequence of the links and the inter-relationship of muscle activation and translation of forces within the body are referred to as the kinetic chain [27]. Each link of this system creates force and energy that are ultimately transferred from the proximal core stabilizing link to the distal peripheral link. When one link is weak or injured, other links compensate. Distal links typically compensate for proximal links, and the added stress and loads result in further injury. For instance, if a patient has weak hip abductors, the knee often has to absorb more of the forces during gait. If the patient also has a tendency to overpronate (flat-foot position), then the forces in the knee are increased. Malalignment of the foot may lead to changes at the knee such as excessive patellofemoral joint pressures and abnormal patellar tracking. Patellar tracking is described as dynamic movement of the kneecap, with its insertion to the tibia and muscle attachment to the quadriceps during extension and flexion of the knee. Hence, proper rehabilitation of patellofemoral joint pain must address factors along the kinetic chain—that is, proximally to the knee (strengthening of the quadriceps, gluteus muscle groups, and hip external rotators) and distally (correcting pronation at the foot) [28].

The role of the therapists

Physical and occupational therapy

Physical therapy is an indispensable part of the treatment continuum. Physical therapists (PTs) and occupational therapists (OTs) use therapeutic exercises, manual techniques, and passive physical modalities to address deficits in flexibility, strength, balance, neuromuscular control, posture, functional mobility, locomotion, and endurance. Both types of therapists also help patients to overcome fear of movement and activity-related pain. Although there is some crossover between the skill sets of PTs and OTs, they possess established core competencies that are fairly universal. PTs specialize in gait training and locomotion, core stability, and activities of daily living such as bed mobility and transfers. They are also experts in the development of aerobic conditioning programs aimed at improving cardiopulmonary health and endurance. OTs typically focus on educating patients regarding proper posture and ergonomics related to upper-limb functional activities such as lifting and computer usage. They address upper-extremity–related activities of daily living including feeding, hygiene, grooming, bathing, and dressing. PTs and OTs also play a primary role in the education of patients, family members, and other caregivers.

PTs and OTs involved in interdisciplinary chronic pain treatment programs must be adept in their ability to assess initial levels of functional ability and then monitor and progressively increase the level and complexity of therapeutic exercises. Most chronic pain patients have secondary impairments in addition to their primary pain-related diagnoses (ie, general inflexibility, deconditioning, myofascial pain, and other postural abnormalities), which are important focuses of treatment. OTs may instruct patients on proper pacing techniques, graded-activity tolerance training, and energy conservation techniques as they apply to physical demands of a task or job.

Recreation therapists

Therapeutic recreation specialists are important members of the rehabilitation team and key team members who help restore patients to previous levels of function that are often lost due to the development of chronic pain. A recreation therapist assessment examines previous patient interests and patient barriers to return to leisure activities. Within a formal program, recreation therapists evaluate and plan leisure activities that serve to promote mental and physical health. Recreation therapists help patients to incorporate strategies learned from various disciplines of multidisciplinary treatment into social and community functions. Application of these techniques in the community and at home (ie, correct biomechanics, pacing, relaxation techniques) leads to the reduction of stress, fear of movement, and depression while fostering a feeling of self-efficacy and confidence. In addition, therapeutic recreation specialists help patients to increase social awareness and promote integration of individuals back into the community.

Treatment modalities used by physical and occupational therapists

Exercise

An exercise regimen specifically tailored to the patient is at the core of a physical or occupational therapy program. Daily exercise is important in maintaining physical health and has been associated with 25% less self-reported musculoskeletal pain (compared with more sedentary control subjects) [29]. In addition, inactivity has been shown to be a predictor of future pain with injury [30]. The therapist usually starts with a prescription from the physician outlining the important diagnoses and the goals of treatment. The therapist then performs his or her own assessment and develops a plan of care. During each session, the therapist works closely with the patient to help alleviate pain and to address physiologic deficits. The goal of treatment is to provide the patient with a home exercise program that can be continued after completion of formal therapy.

Stretching

Until ROM is normalized or near normalized, movement patterns cannot be retrained and strengthening cannot be performed within the physiologic range. Stretching is a key component to restoring normal ROM. When done properly, stretching lengthens tissue including skin, fascia, muscle, and ligaments, thereby increasing overall ROM. Increased ROM decreases contracture, improves functional mobility, and allows the muscles and joints to function properly. ROM exercises vary from passive (in which there is no voluntary muscle contraction and with the application of total external force) to active assisted (in which there is partial contraction and external force) and active (in which there is complete contraction and no external force). In general, most ROM exercises increase blood flow and prevent contracture.

Muscle conditioning

After ROM is normalized, muscle conditioning is addressed because muscles around a joint impact stability, function, and pain. Muscle conditioning comprises three important areas: strength, endurance, and re-education.

Muscle strength is increased through isometric, isotonic, or isokinetic exercises. Isometric strengthening is characterized by contraction of the muscle without change in length or movement. Isometric exercises are typically used in acute pain states such as active inflammation or induced immobilization. Isotonic exercises are those in which muscles contract and the length and movement change but the load remains the same, such as doing a bicep curl with a dumbbell. In contrast, with isokinetic exercise, muscle contracts at a constant angular velocity, such as with a cybex or muscle pulley machine. Muscle strengthening depends on vascularization, energy metabolism, increase in number of myofibrils, and motor unit recruitment. Strengthening muscle tissue results from increasing the load, speed, number, frequency, form, or ROM of the exercise.

Muscle endurance—the ability to sustain and perform repeated contractions—is increased through aerobic activity. Aerobic activity is defined by low-intensity, high-repetition exercise. Walking, running, cycling, and swimming are some examples of aerobic activity used in physical therapy programs. The physiologic changes that occur with aerobic training are numerous and include an increased capillary density around muscle fibers, an increased number of mitochondria, increased activity of mitochondrial enzymes, and increased myoglobin content. Aerobic exercise is also associated with increased levels of endogenous endorphins [31] and enkephalins [32] and may be responsible for an additional antinociceptive or analgesic effect.

Motor re-education may also be simulated with exercise and is often co-ordinated by the therapist as the patient progresses in treatment. Motor re-education involves breaking down a motion into individual chronologic movements. The therapist assists the patient in identifying and then unlearning potentially abnormal movement patterns. Proper posture and retraining of movements are practiced and incorporated into the general strengthening, endurance, and flexibility program [28].

Aquatic therapy

Aerobic and anaerobic exercise can be performed in an aquatic environment. The physiologic advantages of water as a therapeutic medium include thermal conductive properties and high specific heat. The viscosity of water provides resistance for aerobic and strengthening exercises, compressive forces that help to decrease edema, and buoyancy that decreases weight bearing [33]. Therapeutically, aquatic therapy may help in decreasing muscle and joint stiffness and decreasing pain. Hydrostatic forces with immersion in water lead to cardiopulmonary benefits secondary to centralization of blood flow, resulting in increased venous return, stroke volume, cardiac output, and subsequent reflex bradycardia [34,35]. Patients participating in an aquatic therapy program more than 2 days per week as part of a long-term maintenance treatment program demonstrated reduction in pain and improved function [36]. Pool programs are often offered in group settings, providing an added social benefit for the patient.

Mind–body therapy

Mind–body therapy is defined by the National Institutes of Health as an intervention that may "use a variety of techniques designed to facilitate the mind's capacity to affect bodily function and symptoms." Various mind–body treatments may help to improve coordination, decrease abnormal movement patterns, and improve psychologic well-being and include tai chi, body awareness therapy (BAT), and Feldenkrais (FK).

Tai chi, a traditional Chinese mind–body relaxation exercise, consists of approximately 108 intricate exercise sequences performed in a slow, relaxed manner. Tai chi has been found to increase physical and mental health, including physical, social, and emotional function; decrease anxiety; decrease pain perception; and increase flexibility and balance [37–39]. In addition, this mind–body therapy combines the mind with movement to reprogram the nervous system, improve coordination, reduce abnormal motor patterns, and improve physical and emotional health.

BAT and FK are therapies that use patterns of movement to improve flexibility, posture, breathing, and overall function. BAT and FK have been shown to increase body awareness and decrease pain [40]. In addition, BAT and FK improve health-related quality of life and self-efficacy of pain to a higher degree than conventional physiotherapy [41].

Passive modalities

A modality describes any physical agent used to produce a physiologic response in a targeted tissue. Commonly prescribed passive physical modalities for the treatment of acute and chronic pain include cryotherapy, heat, and electrical stimulation. Modalities are initially incorporated into therapy sessions by PTs or OTs, with a goal of educating the patient on appropriate application and use at home. Depending on the specific pain complaint, modalities may be incorporated early in treatment in acute conditions as a means of decreasing local swelling, as analgesia, and to help progression and tolerance of therapies (Boxes 7 and 8, Tables 1 and 2) [42,43]. They are also used as part of a daily treatment regimen (eg, cryotherapy to osteoarthritic knee after exercise, electrical stimulation to low back region during prolonged upright postures) or as a "rescue" treatment for "flare ups."

Electrical stimulation

Transcutaneous electrical nerve stimulation (TENS) and interferential current therapy (ICT) involve the transmission of electrical energy to the peripheral nervous system by way of an external stimulator and conductive gel pads on the skin. TENS is based theoretically on the "gate control theory" proposed by Melzack [44]. TENS stimulates non-nociceptive large afferent A-β fibers "closing" the "gate" of facilitated sensory input, normally "opened" by small-diameter nociceptive C fibers. Electrical stimulation releases endogenous opioids and activates peripherally located α_{2A}-adrenergic receptors [45]. TENS has been shown to be beneficial in acute pain states, reducing the amount of analgesic medication consumed after surgical procedures, and in chronic pain conditions in which it helps to relieve pain and foster patient independence (see Table 2).

Box 7. Cryotherapy

Indication
Acute injury
Muscle spasticity
Osteoarthritis
Minor burns
Arthritis
Bursitis
Acute/chronic pain
Myofascial pain
Contusion inflammation

Effect
Analgesia
Vasoconstriction
Decreases muscle spindle
Decreases nerve conduction
Decreases metabolism
Decreases enzymatic activity
Increases tissue stiffness
Increases viscosity

Example
Ice
Cold pack
Cryotherapy compression unit
Whirlpool bath
Vapo-coolant spray

Contraindication
More than 30 minutes
Ischemia/arterial insufficiency
Raynaud's disease
Impaired sensation
Burns
Cryoglobulinemia
Paroxysmal cold hemoglobinuria
Cold allergy or hypersensitivity

ICT is a variant of TENS that involves the mixing of two unmodulated sine waves with different frequencies (one at 4 kHz and a second within a variable range) to generate frequencies between 4 and 250 Hz. ICT allows for the stimulation of deeper tissues with decreased discomfort. The proposed mechanism of action involves the direct stimulation of muscle

---

Box 8. Heat

Indication
Chronic inflammation
Arthritis
Myofascial pain
Collagen vascular disease
Strains
Sprains
Contracture thrombophlebitis

Effect
Analgesia
Vasodilation, increases blood flow
Increases oxygen and leukocytes
Muscle relaxation
Increases metabolism
Increases capillary permeability
Increases collage extensibility

Contraindication
Acute trauma, inflammation
Bleeding disorders
Edema, scars, impaired sensation
Malignancy
Multiple sclerosis

---

fibers, as opposed to nerve fibers, to achieve improved muscle blood flow and to promote the healing process. Variable frequency helps to prevent adaptation. There is less scientific evidence for the use of ICT compared with TENS.

Manual techniques

Manual techniques may include a number of different approaches for the treatment of acute and chronic pain such as massage, mobilization, and manipulation. Massage therapy has various physiologic effects. The effects of massage can be classified into reflexive and mechanical. Reflexive effects include vasodilatation, resulting in improvement in circulation, endogenous opioid release, and general relaxation. Mechanical effects include assisting venous return and lymphatic drainage, decreasing muscle tightness, and braking adhesions in muscles, tendons, and ligaments. In addition, there is likely a beneficial psychologic effect of massage, which can result in a general sense of well-being. Although massage can produce short-term results, studies have demonstrated mixed results with regard to long-term efficacy

Table 1
Superficial and deep heat therapy

	Composition	Effect	Contraindication
Superficial heat[a]			
Hydrocollator packs	Bags of silicone dioxide heated in stainless steel containers in water 65–90°C	Increases temperature 3.3°C at 1 cm	—
	Applied to body part over towels	Increases temperature 1.3°C at 2 cm [42]	
Paraffin	Paraffin wax and mineral oil in 7:1 ratio heated to 52°C	Increases temperature 5.5°C in forearm subcutaneous tissue	—
	Body part dipped in bath, wax hardens, repeated 7–12 times, then wrapped in plastic and covered by towel	Increases temperature 2.4°C in brachioradialis muscle	
Hydrotherapy			
Whirlpool	Water heated to 40°C (body submersion)	Heats, messages, debrides	—
Hubbard tank	Water heated to 43°C (limb submersion)	Can elevate core temperature depending on surface area	
Fluidotherapy	Hot air blown through medium of dry powder or glass beads at a temperature of 46°C–49°C	Produces temperature of 42°C in hand and joint capsule	—
		Produces temperature of 39.5°C in foot and joint capsule [43]	
Deep heat[b]			
Ultrasound [c]	Electrical current applied to quartz crystal or ceramic	Produces acoustic vibration above the audible range	Heat contraindications
	Heat greatest at areas of impedance: bones > tendon > skin > muscle		Near brain or spine
			Near heart

Table 1 (*continued*)

	Composition	Effect	Contraindication
			Near reproductive organs
			Near pacemakers
			Near tumors
			Gravida or menstruating uterus
			Eyes
			Immature epiphysis
			Arthroplasty

[a] Depth of 0.5–2 cm; amount of heating depends on amount of adipose tissue present.

[b] Depth of 0.5–2 cm; amount of heating depends on amount of adipose tissue present. Heating is by conversion.

[c] Intensity of 0.8–3 W/cm^2; Frequency of 0.8–1 MHz.

[46,47]. Various studies have demonstrated the magnitude of pain reduction as modest [48] and transient between sessions [49]. Diagnostic technique and treatment methods may vary among professional groups (ie, manual therapist, chiropractors, and osteopathic physicians), leading to a difference in treatment outcomes and results of clinical trials [50].

Mobilization involves passive movement of tissue within the limit of joint range. Manipulation may include similar soft tissue techniques in addition to high-velocity techniques whereby forces are generated at a particular joint level beyond physiologic barrier of joint restriction and is more commonly practiced by chiropractic practitioners and osteopathic physicians [51]. Geisser and colleagues [52] found manual therapy with specific adjuvant exercise to be beneficial in treating chronic low back pain with no significant change in function. Others have demonstrated efficacy of spinal manipulation in short-term studies, although the effect size was small compared

Table 2
Transcutaneous electrical nerve stimulation

Tens type	Amplitude/frequency	Indication	Duration	Setting changes
Conventional (low-intensity, high-frequency)	1–2 mA/ 50–100 Hz	Acute pain state	1–20 min for rapid relief 30 min to 2 h for short duration of analgesia Repeat as needed	Increase amplitude or pulse width to avoid adaptation and maintain analgesia
Dense-disperse/ acupuncture-like (high-intensity, low-frequency)	15–20 mA/ 1–5 Hz	Chronic pain state	30 min for short duration 2–6 h for long duration Once daily	Minimal adaptation

with active therapies [53] and placebo [54]. Osteopathic manipulation in a study of subacute low back pain patients demonstrated similar results compared with standard medical care but also used less physical therapy and medications [55].

Pain psychologists

Psychologic factors have been shown to predict long-term disability and contribute to the transition of acute pain to chronic pain [56]. One's cognitions may also impact mood, behavior, and function [57]. Pain psychology assessment and intervention focuses on cognitive and behavioral factors related to pain.

Psychologic interventions are focused on unlearning maladaptive responses and reactions to pain while fostering wellness, improving coping and perceived control, and decreasing catastrophizing. In addition, cognitive interventions focus on fear-avoidance beliefs, a construct that has been closely linked to self-reported disability and physical performance in chronic pain [58,59]. The benefits of cognitive behavioral therapy (CBT) in treating multiple dimensions of chronic pain have been supported by numerous reviews and meta-analyses [60–62]. Coping skills training can be integrated into CBT, focusing on attention-diversion techniques, altering activity patterns, and altering negative-related emotions [63]. The pain psychologists also can contribute to the team as a facilitator of group education classes related to pain and as a guide in relaxation training classes. Formal multidisciplinary and interdisciplinary psychologic treatment may also incorporate family counseling and help to coordinate ongoing psychologic treatment with community counselors at the completion of formal program treatment.

Clinical conditions

This section reviews theoretic issues related to underlying mechanisms of common pain conditions (osteoarthritis [OA], low back pain, myofascial pain, and FM) and principles guiding active physical medicine approaches. In many cases, theses same principles can be applied to other acute and chronic pain conditions.

Osteoarthritis

OA is characterized by an ongoing pathophysiologic cycle. Here, compensatory guarding and pain lead to a loss of ROM, decreased strength and endurance, increasing joint contracture and subsequent development of abnormal posture and motor patterns, joint overload, further joint destruction, and pain. Active therapy is aimed at unloading the joint, improving local muscle condition, and increasing joint and muscle flexibility. Because muscles provide the "dynamic" joint stability during movement, signs of OA, such as osteophytes and capsular thickening, may develop to increase stability when there is muscle dysfunction and dynamic instability. For example, although controversial, it has been proposed that quadriceps dysfunction and weakness may be a risk factor for progression of knee OA [64]. It was found that independent of body weight, knee extensor strength was 18% lower at baseline in women who developed knee OA compared with controls [65]. Studies have shown that exercise programs resulting in increased quadriceps strength and joint position sense reduced pain and improved function. In addition, improvements in quadriceps sensorimotor function resulted in decreased disability in patients who had knee OA and who followed a standard daily exercise regime. In addition to strength, alignment is equally important for dynamic stability and proper functioning. Sharma and colleagues [66] found that quadriceps weakness was not related to progression of knee OA, except in lax and malaligned knees.

A knee orthosis may be helpful when malalignment or instability is present. An orthosis is any externally applied device used to modify structural and functional characteristics of the neuromuscular system [67]. Braces, neoprene sleeves, and foot orthotics have been found to be helpful in increasing stability and in decreasing pain of the knee. Braces and neoprene sleeves have been found to be better than medical treatment alone. Furthermore, braces are more effective than neoprene sleeves in improving stiffness, pain, and function [68]. Dynamic fluoroscopic imaging of braced knees has demonstrated clinically significant distraction between the tibial and femoral condyles [69]. In addition, proprioception, which is commonly reduced in those who have knee OA, is increased with the use of braces [70]. In addition, heel wedges and medial wedge insoles can improve abnormal biomechanics at the foot, ankle, and knee [71]. In addition to foot orthotics, walking aids such as canes, forearm crutches, and walkers are used in those who have OA and gait disturbances. Devices help to unload the joint, improve body mechanics, and decrease pain [72].

Strengthening and endurance exercise relieves symptoms in patients who have mild and moderate OA [73]. Studies have shown that aerobic walking and home-based quadriceps strengthening exercise reduce pain and disability from knee OA [74]. Aerobic exercise only, not strengthening, was found to significantly lower depressive symptoms in high- and low-depressive symptomatology subgroups. Intensity of the aerobic exercise was not a factor. Aerobic cycling at high and low intensities was found to be equally effective in improving functional status, gait, pain, and aerobic capacity with OA of the knee [75]. Thus, exercise appears to moderately decrease pain, increase quadriceps strength, and increase physical function [76]. Exercise has been shown to increase self-efficacy. Self-efficacy is the belief that one has the capabilities to execute the courses of action required to manage prospective situations [77]. In one study, when persons stopped exercising, self-efficacy beliefs declined—only to increase later after resuming exercise [78].

Although exercise is beneficial, it must be actively maintained. Long-term follow-up and compliance of patients who participated in a randomized 3-month intervention showed that the beneficial effects declined with time and disappeared during the 6-month follow-up period [79]. In another study [73], however, significant differences were found in measures of disability, physical performance, and pain after 18 months of exercise in patients who had knee OA. Exercise is also beneficial when combined with the manual therapy or passive movements the therapist uses to increase ROM. A randomized trial [80] compared manual therapy to the knee, hip, foot and ankle, or lumbar spine combined with exercises for lower-extremity strengthening, ROM, and endurance with placebo ultrasound treatment. Significant improvements in pain, the 6-minute walk test, and self-reported function scores were found in the manual therapy plus exercise group compared with the control group. Treatment effects remained at 1-year follow-up.

TENS use and aquatic therapy are also beneficial. TENS use had a positive effect that was greatest with high-intensity burst modes, repeated treatments, and when used for at least 4 weeks [81]. Aquatic therapy has been found to improve aerobic capacity, walk time, physical activity level, and depression in those who have OA [82]. In addition, those who have OA and rheumatoid arthritis have been able to reduce the amount of postural sway (a risk factor for fall) from 18% to 30% with a 6-week aquatic exercise program [33].

Low back pain

Physical therapy approaches for spine-related disorders

A number of active physical therapy treatments for spine-related conditions have demonstrated efficacy in decreasing pain and improving function [83]. The heterogeneous nature of underlying spinal conditions poses a challenge for determining the specific or multiple pain generators involved (ie, disc degeneration, herniation, nerve root compression, facet arthropathy, or sacroiliac dysfunction). From a more mechanical view of low back pain, several subgroups of low back pain exist and may benefit from different exercise treatments. Treatment approaches include cervical and lumbar ROM, stabilization exercises [84], flexion-based exercises (ie, Williams), specific directional preference exercises (ie, McKenzie-based treatment), and neurodynamic techniques. These techniques and underlying theories are reviewed briefly in the following sections, with the understanding of significant overlap and variability between deliveries by therapists.

Stabilization exercises

The concept of lumbar stability has been an area of extensive research for over 30 years. Initial theory was based on an understanding that pain in the spine was the result of gradual degeneration of joints and related soft tissue as a result of microtrauma and poor control of spinal structures, a dynamic process involving static positions and controlled movements [85]. Biomechanical changes of spine stability include postural and motor control that help to reduce tissue strain and provide efficient muscle action [86]. Panjabi [87] classically described a three-component, interdependent system comprising bone and ligamentous structures, muscles, and the neural control system. An important focus of spine stability for low back pain includes assessment and strengthening of core muscle groups, controlling intersegmental stability, and restoring motion [88].

A basic individualized physical therapy approach includes stretching tight or contracted muscles, activating inhibited muscles, and improving core strength. Exercises are commonly targeted on retraining the multifidus (back muscle) and transverses abdominus (a deep abdominal muscle) along with supplemented exercises for the pelvic floor and breathing control [21]. Therapists help to train patients to contract these muscles independently from more superficial muscles. As the patient progresses through core strengthening, balance and conditioning are incorporated into the exercise program. These exercises can be facilitated with the use of an exercise or medicine ball, balance boards, theraband elastic strips, and an air-filled plastic disc with adjustable inflations [89]. Research has suggested that stability exercises may prevent recurrence of pain and improve function in patients compared with control groups [84,90].

Directional preference

The concept of centralization, recognized and popularized by McKenzie [91], is based on the concept by which pain radiating from the cervical, thoracic, or lumbar spine is sequentially abolished, neurologic symptoms are decreased [92], or a reduction of symptoms is noted [93,94] distally to proximally in the affected limb or body region in response to spinal positions or maneuvers (ie, extension, flexion, side bending). Centralization phenomena can be reliably assessed, and because of its association with more favorable clinical outcomes (physical therapy and lumbar surgery), it can be used to guide treatment in selected patients [95–97].

Peripheralization, the opposite response, involves the distal spread of pain into the limb with similar positioning. Noncentralization has been shown to be a more reliable predictor of poorer outcomes in physical therapy and surgery. In the sole trial involving subacute pain [98], those who underwent a graded-activity program returned to work more quickly, had fewer absences during the next 2 years, and had improved back mobility and fitness.

Neurodynamic therapy

Neurodynamic therapy is based on the concept of altered mechanosensitivity of the damaged neurogenic tissue. It is based on a more comprehensive functional understanding of the peripheral and central nervous system plasticity. Classically, this is represented clinically by a positive straight-leg raise, identifying the possible presence of perineuritis. Maitland [99] more formally described this as the slump test (or seated straight-leg raise), which incorporates cervical flexion and ankle dorsiflexion as a means of assessing mechanosensitivity of neural structures within the spinal vertebral canal. Peripheral nerves may become pain generators due to related innervated connective tissue or injury processes along the nerve myelin sheath. Butler [100] described abnormal impulse-generating sites as areas of injury along the central nervous system where ion channels accumulate, leading to abnormal firing. Therapy is focused peripherally at decreasing the firing of abnormal impulse-generating sites by improving mobility of the nerve by decreasing tension or pressure along the perineural structures.

Exercise

Exercise benefits in low back pain treatment have been demonstrated with regard to improved muscle performance, strength, and endurance [59,101]. General exercise guidelines may be useful in developing an individual treatment program for acute and chronic pain conditions. The American College of Sports Medicine proposed three areas of focus, including (1) muscle strengthening, (2) flexibility training, and (3) cardiovascular endurance as discussed earlier in this article [102]. Exercise-based treatments may help to promote wellness rather than illness behavior [103] and empower patients to take a more active role in their progress toward improved function [59,104]. Meta-analysis and reviews have shown exercise-based treatment to be more effective at decreasing pain and improving function with chronic low back pain [105] compared with reviews of acute low back pain [106]. Of interest, a systematic review of exercise therapy concluded that specific back exercises should not be recommended for acute or chronic pain but that exercise in general may be beneficial as part of an active rehabilitation program [106]. Keller and colleagues [107] examined lumbar paraspinal muscle density—an indication of muscle strength—in patients who underwent lumbar fusion compared with a nonsurgical group. The nonsurgical group participated in a low-intensity exercise and cognitive behavioral interventional program. The exercise and cognitive intervention group demonstrated significant improvement in lumbar strength (increased by 30%) at 1 year compared with surgical counterparts. Lumbar fusion patients demonstrated a 10% reduction in muscle density, whereas the exercise group's muscle density remained unchanged. Other studies have also suggested that activity in general may itself be therapeutic in reducing pain and improving psychosocial functioning [108,109].

Myofascial pain syndrome

Myofascial pain syndrome (MPS) is characterized by tenderness in the muscle, characteristic pain referral patterns, and restriction of motion [110]. MPS may be a primary source of pain or be present as part of a more complicated multifactorial pain condition. Trigger points are discrete, focal, hyperirritable spots located in a taut band of skeletal muscle that are painful on compression and may produce referred pain, referred tenderness, motor and or autonomic dysfunction, and autonomic dysfunction. Myofascial trigger points (MTrPs) may be classified as active or latent. Latent trigger points are tender to palpation and may be associated with restricted ROM and stiffness but are not associated with spontaneous complaints of pain. MTrPs are commonly found in postural muscles including the neck, shoulders, and pelvic girdle and in the upper trapezius, scalene, levator scapulae, quadratus lumborum, and lumbosacral muscles. MTrP may develop or be aggravated by acute tissue trauma, repetitive microtrauma, muscle deconditioning, postural abnormalities, poor sleep, or metabolic abnormalities (ie, vitamin deficiencies, hypothyroidism [111]). Occupational and recreational activities often precipitate or aggravate MPS. Common workplace activities such as holding a telephone receiver between the ear and shoulder, prolonged bending over a table, sitting in chairs with poor back support, improper height of arm rests and computer work stations, and moving boxes using improper body mechanics [112] may lead to musculoskeletal dysfunction and MPS (Table 3).

Diagnosis of MPS is primarily based on clinical findings. Clinically, confirmation of MPS is not related to any specific laboratory tests (eg, imaging studies, electromyography, or muscle biopsy). Assessment of posture, body mechanics, dynamic joint function, and palpation of MTrPs may help to confirm the diagnosis. In assessing active MTrPs, one palpates across muscle fibers, and feels for a "rope like" nodularity of tight muscle. These discrete areas may reproduce characteristic pain-referral patterns usually

Table 3
Soft tissue pain

Characteristic	Myofascial pain	Fibromyalgia
Clinical sign	Local tenderness	Local tenderness or diffuse pain for 3 mo
	Referred pain pattern	Tender points
	Trigger points	11 of 18 symmetric tender points are positive
	Pain in taut band of muscle	
	Local twitch response	
	"Jump sign"	
Sex predominance	Male = female	Female > male
Location	Occur in any muscle	Specific locations: fat pad, epicondyle, joint, muscle insertion site, muscle
	Asymmetric	Symmetric
Associated factors	Acute tissue trauma	Insidious cause of pain
	Repetitive microtrauma	Increase in pain sensitivity
	Muscle deconditioning	Sleep disturbance
	Postural abnormalities	Increase in catastrophizing
	Sensitized nerve foci	Decreased serotonin production

traveling in a proximal to distal direction. There may be a local "twitch response," characterized by a palpable and visible reflex contraction of involved muscle. A "jump sign" is a pain-related withdrawal reflex secondary to applied pressure to a painful MTrP.

Although the physical examination is sensitive and specific in diagnosing MPS, research has demonstrated fine-needle electromyographic findings characteristic of the disorder and may help to develop mechanistic strategies for pharmacologic and nonpharmacologic treatment. Abnormal acetylcholine release at the motor end plate, and end plate noise is more frequent in MTrPs than at end plates outside of the zone or MTrPs. End plate noise is characteristic but not diagnostic of MTrPs and may be increased in any situation in which there is a mechanical, chemical, or other noxious stimuli. With sustained acetylcholine release, sarcomeres shorten, which produces a "contraction knot." This increase in sarcomere activity results in an increase in energy consumption and a relative reduction in circulation, creating localized hypoxia and ischemia. Pronociceptive substances such as bradykinin, serotonin, and histamine are in turn released, sensitizing afferents and producing local tenderness. Central convergence and facilitation at the level of the dorsal horn leads to referred pain in adjacent myotomes and to expansion of receptive fields. Increased neuronal excitability at the level of the dorsal horn leads to the release of substance P and glutamate key players in the development and maintenance of central sensitization.

The autonomic nervous system may also be activated by neurovasoreactive substances (ie, bradykinin, substance P, serotonin, and histamine). With autonomic nervous system activation, more acetylcholine is released. Audette and colleagues [37], in a study of dry-needle treatment of MTrPs, found that bilateral motor unit activation was produced with unilateral needle stimulation of the symptomatic MTrP. Contralateral or mirror-image electromyographic activity may support the concept of abnormal central nervous system processing of sensory input at the level of the spinal cord as a key perpetuator of pain and muscle dysfunction. Clinically, ongoing psychologic stress, maladaptive posture, and elevated muscle tension may also contribute to the muscle pain dysfunction cycle [113].

Effective treatment of MPS focuses on pharmacologic and nonpharmacologic treatments including physical and occupational therapy, exercise, ergonomic assessment, relaxation and stress reduction training. Physical and occupational treatment goals include reducing pain, restoring ROM, and improving function. MTrP muscles fatigue more rapidly and recover more slowly. Therapies involve a graded stabilization and strengthening program. When strengthening is done too early, there is the risk for overload and compensation of other muscles, which may develop MTrP. In addition, physical and occupational therapy are important in helping to reduce fear of movement and are incorporated in a gradually progressive submaximal exercise program, helping the patient to gain confidence in independent movements. Muscle-release techniques and other self-management approaches are commonly included. Overall, stretching is the basis of all exercise programs for MPS because it is vital to reset the muscle fiber length. Aerobic exercises have been found to increase endogenous pain control, improve mood, have additive effects with physical therapy, and prevent recurrence of MPS.

Modalities, such as the spray and stretch technique, involve the therapist passively stretching the target muscle while simultaneously applying a local soft tissue coolant. Chemicals such as dichlorodifluoromethane-trichloro-monofluoromethane or ethyl chloride spray produce a drop in skin temperature and temporary anesthesia, theoretically blocking the spinal stretch reflex and sensation of pain centrally. The muscle may then be passively stretched toward its normal length, inactivating trigger points, relieving spasm, and reducing referred pain.

Another commonly used modality, TENS, may be used for acute or chronic myofascial pain; see the earlier section "Electrical stimulation." High-frequency, high-intensity TENS has been shown to reduce pain in MPS. High-power ultrasound applied to the trigger points before stretching was found to be more effective than conventional ultrasound and to significantly decrease the length of therapy [114]. One study looked at the immediate effects of various physical therapeutic modalities on cervical myofascial pain and trigger-point sensitivity and found that hot pack plus active ROM plus ICT plus myofascial release technique was more effective for easing MTrP pain and increasing cervical ROM [115] than hot pack plus active ROM plus stretch and spray plus TENS, which was more effective than hot pack plus active ROM plus stretch and spray.

Interventional treatments such as trigger point injections and acupuncture have been found to be effective in treating MTrP. In comparative studies, dry needling was found to be as effective as injecting an anesthetic solution such as procaine or lidocaine. Postinjection soreness, however, was more intense and of longer duration than the soreness with lidocaine. In one study, 58% of subjects reported verbal rating scores (VRS) of 0 on a 0 to 10 scale immediately after trigger-point injection; 42% had minimal pain scores (1 to 2 on a 10-point VRS) [116]; however, overall pain relief did not differ, supporting the theory that mechanical disruption of the muscle fibers and the increase in blood flow is important in relieving pain. Porta [117], in a single-center randomized study, reported a greater reduction in pain in patients who had chronic MPS injected with botulinum toxin type A (BTX-A) compared with steroid. Pain-reduction gains continued at 60 days in the BTX-A group but decreased in the steroid-treated patients. BTX-A has been studied in other MPS-related disorders, showing efficacy in cervicogenic pain [118] and mixed outcomes with headache disorders [119–121]. BTX-A has been compared with dry needling and lidocaine trigger-point injections and has not been found to be cost-effective [63].

Fibromyalgia

FM syndrome (FMS), another common musculoskeletal pain disorder, may share some common characteristics with MPS and may coexist in patients; however, these disorders may remain distinct, although there may be significant sign and symptom overlap (see Table 3). FMS is characterized by widespread musculoskeletal pain (at least 3 months) and stiffness, with symmetrically distributed tender points (TPs) and associated symptoms (ie, irritable bowel/bladder syndrome, dysautonomia, cognitive and endocrine dysfunction, dizziness, cold intolerance, or mood disorder) [122].

Recent studies support evidence of central changes in brain processing [123] and neurochemical abnormalities (elevated excitatory neurotransmitter substance P [124], nitric oxide [125], and amino acids [126]) as possible mediators of peripheral and central sensitization.

TPs, distinguished from MTrPs associated with MPS, are characterized by eliciting pain with at least 4 kg of pressure to at least 11 or 18 muscle tendon sites, based on common research criteria [127]. Reported prevalence rates of FM are approximately 2% in the United States, including 3.4% of women and 0.5% of men [127]. FMS patients may have lowered mechanical and thermal pain thresholds and psychologic factors including increased levels of catastrophizing [128].

The comprehensive treatment of FM involves a balance between rational pharmacologic treatments, exercise, physical and occupational therapy, and patient education. This multidisciplinary approach has demonstrated successful treatment outcomes such as decreased depression, self-reported pain behaviors, observed pain behaviors, and myalgia scores [129].

FM was once considered a "nonrestorative sleep syndrome," and evidence exists that patients who have FM do not obtain adequate amounts of restorative non–rapid eye movement sleep [130], which may result from disorders of serotonin metabolism. Thus, encouraging proper sleep hygiene and restoring proper levels of serotonin and non–rapid eye movement sleep is important in reducing pain and fatigue.

Physical medicine approaches to managing FMS include a comprehensive program incorporating a range of pharmacologic and nonpharmacologic strategies including active physical therapy, exercise, cognitive and behavioral treatments, and patient education (Box 9) [131]. A recent study identified clusters of patients based on severity of TP tenderness, affective distress (depression and anxiety), and psychologic traits (sense of self-efficacy and catastrophizing) and may help to individually classify the level of clinical intervention needed [132].

Pharmacologic management is an important aspect in the treatment of FM and focuses on decreasing pain, improving mood, and restoring quality sleep. Medicines are focused on modulating levels of serotonin, norepinephrine, and substance P. The tricyclic antidepressants amitriptyline and cyclobenzaprine, taken at night [133], and tramadol [134] have been found to be

---

Box 9. Stepwise fibromyalgia management

Step 1
- Confirm the diagnosis.
- Explain the condition.
- Evaluate and treat comorbid illnesses such as mood disturbance and primary sleep disturbances.

Step 2
- Initiate trial of low-dose tricyclic antidepressant or cyclobenzaprine.
- Begin cardiovascular fitness exercise program.
- Refer patient for CBT or combine with exercise.

Step 3
- Make a specialty referral (eg, rheumatologist, physiatrist, psychiatrist, pain management).
- Conduct trials with selective serotonin reuptake inhibitor, serotonin and norepinephrine reuptake inhibitor, or tramadol.
- Consider a combination-medication trial or anticonvulsant.

---

effective. Selective serotonin reuptake inhibitors are helpful, and fluoxetine has been found to decrease fatigue, depression, and pain [135]. Newer pharmacologic agents that include serotonin norepinephrine dual-reuptake inhibitors, including venlafaxine and duloxetine, and pregabalin, an anticonvulsant and calcium channel modulator, may help to decrease central sensitization and have demonstrated efficacy in decreasing pain and improving sleep [131,136,137].

The pain and fatigue reported by individuals who have FM results in a relative sedentary lifestyle and, hence, a decrease in the fitness level of skeletal muscles. Low-intensity aerobic exercise regimens are effective in reducing the number of TPs in total myalgic scores and reducing TP tenderness, and improving aerobic capacity, physical function, subjective well-being, and self-efficacy. Aerobic exercise also has been found to be better than stretching in decreasing depression, pain, and the emotional aspects and mental health domains of the Medical Outcomes Study Short Form Survey (SF-36) [138].

FMS patients may have difficulty tolerating general exercise programs due to fatigue and muscle sensitivity. Gowans and deHueck [139] recommended that (1) exercise be initiated below the patient's capacity and increased gradually, (2) patients be aware of tolerable short-term increase in pain and fatigue after initiating exercise, and (3) capacity to exercise be increased over time, with similar or lower levels of pain.

Pool therapy has been found to improve cardiovascular capacity, walking time, number of days of feeling good, self-reported physical impairment, pain, anxiety, depression, and daytime fatigue in those who have FM [140].

CBT has been found to improve pain, fatigue, mood, and function in FMS [141]. In general, CBT includes three treatment components (educational phase, skills training, and application phase) focusing on changes in negative perceptions of pain, improved coping and relaxation strategy training, and relapse prevention [142]. Greater benefits of CBT may be found when used adjunctively with exercise and other active treatments [143].

Multidisciplinary tertiary center-based outpatient programs have also been found to be beneficial in patients who have FM by incorporating structured multimodal treatment (pharmacologic management, physical therapy and exercise, psychologic treatment, and education) [144]. A recent review found that multidisciplinary approaches were effective for decreasing pain, decreasing impact of FMS, and increasing self-efficacy and walk time [145]. Pfeiffer and colleagues [146] examined a 1.5-day multidisciplinary treatment program that incorporated educational and self-management sessions, physical and occupational therapy, and medical management and demonstrated a positive effect on impact of illness in FMS patients who did and did not have concomitant depression. In general, compared with pharmacologic treatment, nonpharmacologic treatment appears to be more efficacious in improving self-report of FMS symptoms than pharmacologic treatment alone [141].

Summary

A physical medicine and rehabilitation approach to acute and chronic pain syndromes includes a wide spectrum of treatment focus. Whether assessing or treating acute or chronic pain syndromes, management should include a biopsychosocial approach. Assessment may include a focused joint and functional examination including more global areas of impairment (ie, gait, balance, and endurance) and disability. More complicated multidimensional chronic pain conditions may require the use of a more collaborative continuum of multidisciplinary and interdisciplinary treatment approaches. Regardless of the scope of care that each individual patient requires, treatment options may include active physical therapy, rational polypharmacy, CBT, and the use of passive modalities. Treatment goals generally emphasize achieving analgesia, improving psychosocial functioning, and reintegration of recreational or leisure pursuits (ie, community activities and sports). Progress in all therapies necessitates close monitoring by the health care provider and necessitates ongoing communication between members of the treatment team. Although this article focuses on diagnoses related to acute and chronic low back pain, OA, and musculoskeletal disorders, assessment and treatment recommendations may be generalized to most other pain conditions.

References

[1] World Health Organization. International classification of impairments, disabilities, and handicaps. Geneva (Switzerland): WHO; 1980.
[2] Boon H, Verhoef M, O'Hara D, et al. From parallel practice to integrative health care: a conceptual framework. BMC Health Serv Res 2004;4:1–5.
[3] Wolf CJ, Costigan M. Transcriptional and posttranslational plasticity and the generation of inflammation. Proc Natl Acad Sci U S A 1999;96:7723–30.
[4] Price DD. Psychological and neural mechanisms of the affective dimension of pain. Science 2000;288:1769–72.
[5] Engel GL. The need for a new medical model: a challenge for biomedical science. Science 1977;196:129–36.
[6] Frey SG, Fordyce WE. Behavioral rehabilitation of the chronic pain patient. Annu Rev Rehabil 1983;3:32–63.
[7] Turk DC, Meichenbaum D, Genest M. Pain and behavioral medicine: a cognitive-behavioral perspective. New York: Guildford Press; 1983.
[8] Anonymous. Guide for the uniform data set for medical rehabilitation (adult FIM). Version 4.0. Buffalo (NY): State University of New York at Buffalo; 1993.
[9] Fordyce WE. Behavioral methods for chronic pain and illness. St. Louis (MO): Mosby; 1976.
[10] Keefe FJ, Block AR, Williams RB Jr, et al. Behavioral treatment of chronic low back pain: clinical outcome and individual differences in pain relief. Pain 1981;11(2):221–31.
[11] Turk DC, Wack JT, Kerns RD. An empirical examination of the "pain-behavior" construct. J Behav Med 1985;8:119–30.
[12] McCahon S, Strong J, Sharry R, et al. Self-report and pain behavior among patients with chronic pain. Clin J Pain 2005;21(3):223–31.
[13] Waddell G, Main CJ. Illness behavior. Edinburgh (UK): Churchill Livingstone; 1998.
[14] Fishbain DA, Rosomoff HL, Cutler RB, et al. Secondary gain concept: a review of the scientific evidence. Clin J Pain 1995;11:6–21.
[15] Fishbain DA, Cutler RB, Rosomoff HL, et al. Is there a relationship between nonorganic physical findings (Waddell Signs) and secondary gain/malingering? Clin J Pain 2004;20(6):399–408.
[16] Balzini L, Vannucchi L, Benvenuti F, et al. Clinical characteristics of flexed posture in elderly women. J Am Geriatr Soc 2003;51(10):1419–26.
[17] Al-Eisa E, Egan D, Deluzio K, et al. Effects of pelvic asymmetry and low back pain on trunk kinematics during sitting: a comparison with standing. Spine 2006;31:E135–43.
[18] Jull GA, Janda V. Muscles and motor control in low back pain: assessment and management. New York: Churchill Livingstone; 1987.
[19] Janda V. Physical therapy of the cervical and thoracic spine. New York: Churchill Livingstone; 1998.
[20] Janda V. Muscles and motor control in cervicogenic disorders: assessment and management. New York: Churchill Livingstone; 1994.
[21] Richardson CG. Therapeutic exercises for spinal stabilization and low back pain: scientific bases and clinical approach. Edinburgh (UK): Churchill Livingstone; 1999.
[22] Laasonen EM. Atrophy of sacrospinal muscle groups in patients with chronic, diffusely radiating lumbar back pain. Neuroradiology 1984;26(1):9–13.
[23] Bergmark A. Stability of the lumbar spine. A study in mechanical engineering. Acta Orthop Scand Suppl 1989;230:1–54.

[24] Radebold A, Cholewicki J, Polzhofer GK, et al. Impaired postural control of the lumbar spine is associated with delayed muscle response times in patients with chronic idiopathic low back pain. Spine 2001;26:724–30.
[25] Hodges PW, Richardson CA. Inefficient muscular stabilization of the lumbar spine associated with low back pain: a motor control evaluation of transverse abdominis. Spine 1996; 80:1005–12.
[26] Esquenazi A, Hirai B. Assessment of gait and orthotic prescription. Phys Med Rehabil Clin N Am 1991;2:473–85.
[27] Kibler WB. Determining the extent of the functional deficit. In: Herring SA, Press JM, editors. Functional rehabilitation of sports and musculoskeletal injuries. 1st edition. Gaithersburg (MD): Aspen Publication; 1998. p. 16–9.
[28] Brukner P, Kahn K. Clinical sports medicine. 2nd edition. McGraw Hill; 2001.
[29] Bruce B, Fries JF, Lubeck DP. Aerobic exercise and its impact on musculoskeletal pain in older adults: a 14 year prospective, longitudinal study. Arthritis Res Ther 2005;7(6): R1263–70.
[30] Taimela S, Diederich C, Hubsch M, et al. The role of physical exercise and inactivity in pain recurrence and absenteeism from work after active outpatient rehabilitation for recurrent or chronic low back pain: a follow-up study. Spine 2000;25(14):1809–16.
[31] Farrell PA, Gates WK, Maksud MG, et al. Increases in plasma beta-endorphin/beta-lipotropin immunoreactivity after treadmill running in humans. J Appl Physiol 1982;52(5): 1245–9.
[32] Grossman A, Sutton JR. Endorphins: what are they? How are they measured? What is their role in exercise? Med Sci Sports Exerc 1985;17(1):74–81.
[33] Suomi R, Collier D. Effects of arthritis exercise programs on functional fitness and perceived activities of daily living measures in older adults with arthritis. Arch Phys Med Rehabil 2003;84(11):1589–94.
[34] Choukroun M, Kays C, Varene P. Effects of water temperature on pulmonary volumes in immersed human subjects. Respir Physiol 1989;75:255–66.
[35] Anstey K, Roskell C. Hydrotherapy: detrimental or beneficial to the respiratory system? Physiotherapy 2000;86:5–12.
[36] Ariyoshi M, Sonoda K, Nagata K, et al. Efficacy of aquatic exercises for patients with low-back pain. Kurume Med J 1999;46(2):91–6.
[37] Audette J, Wang F, Smith HS. Bilateral activation of motor unit potentials with unilateral needle stimulation of active myofascial trigger points. Am J Phys Med Rehabil 2004;83: 368–74.
[38] Ross MC, Bohannon AS, Davis DC, et al. The effects of a short-term exercise program on movement, pain, and mood in the elderly. Results of a pilot study. J Holist Nurs 1999;17(2): 139–47.
[39] Song R, Lee EO, Lam P, et al. Effects of tai chi exercise on pain, balance, muscle strength, and perceived difficulties in physical functioning in older women with osteoarthritis: a randomized clinical trial. J Rheumatol 2003;30(9):2039–44.
[40] Gard G. Body awareness therapy for patients with fibromyalgia and chronic pain. Disabil Rehabil 2005;27(12):725–8.
[41] Malmgren-Olsson EB, Branholm IB. A comparison between three physiotherapy approaches with regard to health-related factors in patients with non-specific musculoskeletal disorders. Disabil Rehabil 2002;24(6):308–17.
[42] Lehmann JF, Silverman DR, Baum BA, et al. Temperature distributions in the human thigh, produced by infrared, hot pack and microwave applications. Arch Phys Med Rehabil 1966;47(5):291–9.
[43] Borrell RM, Parker R, Henley EJ, et al. Comparison of in vivo temperatures produced by hydrotherapy, paraffin wax treatment, and fluidotherapy. Phys Ther 1980; 60(10):1273–6.
[44] Melzack R, Wall P. Pain mechanisms: a new theory. Sci Justice 1965;150:971–9.

[45] King EW, Audette K, Athman GA, et al. Transcutaneous electrical nerve stimulation activates peripherally located alpha-2A adrenergic receptors. Pain 2005;115(3):364–73.

[46] Ernst E. Massage therapy for low back pain. J Pain Symptom Manage 1999;17:65–9.

[47] Furlan A, Brosseau L, Imamura M, et al. Massage for low back pain. A systematic review. Cochrane Database Syst Rev 2002;2:CD001929.

[48] Cherkin DC, Eisenberg D, Sherman KJ, et al. Randomized trial comparing traditional Chinese medical acupuncture, therapeutic massage, and self-care education for chronic low back pain. Arch Intern Med 2001;161(8):1081–8.

[49] Hernandez-Reif M, Field T, Krasnegor J, et al. Lower back pain is reduced and range of motion increased after massage therapy. Int J Neurosci 2001;106:131–45.

[50] Van de Veen E, De Vet H, Pool J, et al. Variance in manual treatment of nonspecific low back pain between orthomanual physicians, manual therapists, and chiropractors. J Manipulative Physiol Ther 2005;28:108–16.

[51] Greenman P. Principles of manual medicine. 2nd edition. Baltimore (MD): Williams and Wilkins; 1996.

[52] Geisser M, Wiggert E, Haig A, et al. A randomized, controlled trial of manual therapy and specific adjuvant exercise for chronic low back pain. Clin J Pain 2005;21:463–70.

[53] Assendelft WJ, Morton SC, Yu EI, et al. Spinal manipulative therapy for low back pain. A meta-analysis of effectiveness relative to other therapies. Ann Intern Med 2003;138(11):871–81.

[54] Ferreira ML, Ferreira PH, Latimer J, et al. Does spinal manipulative therapy help people with chronic low back pain? Aust J Physiother 2002;48(4):277–84.

[55] Andersson GB, Lucente T, Davis AM, et al. A comparison of osteopathic spinal manipulation with standard care for patients with low back pain. N Engl J Med 1999;341(19):1426–31.

[56] Burton AK, Battie MC, Main CJ. The relative importance of biomechanical and psychosocial factors in low back injuries. In: Karwowski W, Marras W, editors. The occupational ergonomics handbook. Boca Raton (FL): CRC Press; 1999. p. 1127–38.

[57] Linton SJ. A review of psychological risk factors in back and neck pain. Spine 2000;25(9):1148–56.

[58] Crombez G, Vlaeyen JWS, Heuts PH. Pain-related fear is more disabling than pain itself: evidence on the role of pain-related fear in chronic back pain disability. Pain 1999;80:920–9.

[59] Mannion AF, Junge A, Taimela S, et al. Active therapy for chronic low back pain: part 3. Factors influencing self-rated disability and its change following therapy. Spine 2001;26(8):920–9.

[60] McCracken LM, Turk D. Behavioral and cognitive behavioral treatment for chronic pain: outcome, predictors of outcome, and treatment process. Spine 2002;22:2564–73.

[61] Morley S, Eccleston C, Williams A. Systematic review and meta-analysis of randomized trials of cognitive behavior therapy and behavior therapy for chronic pain in adults, excluding headache. Pain 1999;80:1–13.

[62] van Tulder MV, Ostelo R, Vlaeyen JW, et al. Behavioral treatment for low back pain: a systematic review within the framework of the Chochrane Back Review Group. Spine 2001;26:270–81.

[63] Kamanli A, Kaya A, Ardicoglu O, et al. Comparison of lidocaine injection, botulinum toxin injection, and dry needling to trigger points in myofascial pain syndrome. Rheumatol Int 2005;25(8):604–11.

[64] Slemenda C, Brandt KD, Heilman DK, et al. Quadriceps weakness and osteoarthritis of the knee. Ann Intern Med 1997;127(2):97–104.

[65] Slemenda C, Heilman DK, Brandt KD, et al. Reduced quadriceps strength relative to body weight: a risk factor for knee osteoarthritis in women? Arthritis Rheum 1998;41(11):1951–9.

[66] Sharma L, Song J, Felson DT, et al. The role of knee alignment in disease progression and functional decline in knee osteoarthritis. JAMA 2001;286(2):188–95.

[67] Redford J, Basmajian J, Trautman P. Orthotics: clinical practice and rehabilitation technology. New York: Churchill Livingstone; 1995.

[68] Brouwer RW, Jakma TS, Verhagen AP, et al. Braces and orthoses for treating osteoarthritis of the knee. Cochrane Database Syst Rev 2005;1:CD004020.

[69] Komistek RD, Dennis DA, Northcut EJ, et al. An in vivo analysis of the effectiveness of the osteoarthritic knee brace during heel-strike of gait. J Arthroplasty 1999;14(6):738–42.

[70] Birmingham TB, Kramer JF, Kirkley A, et al. Knee bracing after ACL reconstruction: effects on postural control and proprioception. Med Sci Sports Exerc 2001;33(8):1253–8.

[71] Ogata K, Yasunaga M, Nomiyama H. The effect of wedged insoles on the thrust of osteoarthritic knees. Int Orhop 1997;21(5):308–12.

[72] Van der Esch M, Heijmans M, Dekker J. Factors contributing to possession and use of walking aids among persons with rheumatoid arthritis and osteoarthritis. Arthritis Rheum 2003;49(6):838–42.

[73] Ettinger WHJ, Burns R, Messier SP, et al. A randomized trial comparing aerobic exercise and resistance exercise with a health education program in older adults with knee osteoarthritis. The Fitness Arthritis and Seniors Trial (FAST). JAMA 1997;277(1):25–31.

[74] Roddy E, Zhang W, Doherty M. Aerobic walking or strengthening exercise for osteoarthritis of the knee? A systematic review. Ann Rheum Dis 2005;64(4):544–8.

[75] Mangione KK, McCully K, Gloviak A, et al. The effects of high-intensity and low-intensity cycle ergometry in older adults with knee osteoarthritis. J Gerontol A Biol Sci Med Sci 2000; 54(4):M184–90.

[76] Van Baar ME, Dekker J, Oostendorp RA, et al. The effectiveness of exercise therapy in patients with osteoarthritis of the hip or knee: a randomized clinical trial. J Rheumatol 1998; 25(12):2432–9.

[77] Baron RA, Byrne D, Branscombe NR. Social psychology. 11th edition (MyPsychLab Series). Boston: Allyn & Bacon; 2005.

[78] McAuley E, Lox C, Duncan TE. Long-term maintenance of exercise, self-efficacy, and physiological change in older adults. J Gerontol A Biol Sci Med Sci 1993;48(4):218–24.

[79] Van Baar ME, Dekker J, Oostendorp RA, et al. Effectiveness of exercise in patients with osteoarthritis of hip or knee: nine months' follow up. Ann Rheum Dis 2001;60(12):1123–30.

[80] Deyle GD, Henderson NE, Matekel RL, et al. Effectiveness of manual physical therapy and exercise in osteoarthritis of the knee. A randomized, controlled trial. Ann Intern Med 2000; 132(3):173–81.

[81] Osiri M, Welch V, Brosseau L, et al. Transcutaneous electrical nerve stimulation for knee osteoarthritis. Cochrane Database Syst Rev 2000;4:CD002823.

[82] Bunning RD, Materson RS. A rational program of exercise for patients with osteoarthritis. Semin Arthritis Rheum 1991;21(3 Suppl):33–43.

[83] Malmivaara A, Hakkinen U, Aro T, et al. The treatment of acute low back pain—bed rest, exercises, or ordinary activity? N Engl J Med 1995;332:351–5.

[84] O'Sullivan PB, Phyty GD, Twomey LT, et al. Evaluation of specific stabilizing exercise in the treatment of chronic low back pain with radiologic diagnosis of spondylolysis or spondylolisthesis. Spine 1997;22(24):2959–67.

[85] Barr KP, Griggs M, Cadby T. Lumbar stabilization: core concepts and current literature, part 1. Am J Phys Med Rehabil 2005;84(6):473–80.

[86] Sahrman SA. Does postural assessment contribute to patient care? J Orthop Sports Phys Ther 2002;32(8):376–9.

[87] Panjabi MM. The stabilizing system of the spine. Part I. Function, dysfunction, adaptation, and enhancement. J Spinal Disord 1992;5(4):383–9 [discussion: 397].

[88] Cholewicki J, McGill SM. Lumbar posterior ligament involvement during extremely heavy lifts estimated from fluoroscopic measurements. J Biomech 1992;25(1):17–28.

[89] Akuthota V, Nadler SF. Core strengthening. Arch Phys Med Rehabil 2004;85(3, Suppl 1): S86–92.

[90] Hides J. Paraspinal mechanism and support of the lumbar spine. Edinburgh (UK): Churchill Livingstone; 2004.

[91] McKenzie R. The lumbar spine. Mechanical diagnosis and therapy. Waikanae (New Zealand): Spinal Publications; 1981.

[92] Fritz JM, Delitto A, Vignovic M, et al. Interrater reliability of judgments of the centralization phenomenon and status change during movement testing in patients with low back pain. Arch Phys Med Rehabil 2000;81(1):57–61.

[93] Delitto A, Cibulka MT, Erhard RE, et al. Evidence for use of an extension-mobilization category in acute low back syndrome: a prescriptive validation pilot study. Phys Ther 1993;73(4):216–28.

[94] Erhard RE, Delitto A, Cibulka MT. Relative effectiveness of an extension program and a combined program of manipulation and flexion and extension exercises in patients with acute low back syndrome. Phys Ther 1994;74(12):1093–100.

[95] Werneke M, Hart DL. Centralization phenomenon as a prognostic factor for chronic low back pain and disability. Spine 2001;26(7):758–64 [discussion: 765].

[96] Wetzel FT, Donelson R. The role of repeated end-range/pain response assessment in the management of symptomatic lumbar discs. Spine 2003;3(2):146–54.

[97] Aina A, May S, Clare H. The centralization phenomenon of spinal symptoms—a systematic review. Man Ther 2004;9(3):134–43.

[98] Lindstrom I, Ohlund C, Eek C, et al. Mobility, strength, and fitness after a graded activity program for patients with subacute low back pain. A randomized prospective clinical study with a behavioral therapy approach. Spine 1992;17(6):641–52.

[99] Maitland G. The slump test: examination and treatment. Aust J Physiother 1985;31:215–9.

[100] Butler D. Sensitive nervous system. Adelaide (Australia): Noigroup Publications; 2000.

[101] Liddle SD, Baxter GD, Gracey JH. Exercise and chronic low back pain: what works? Pain 2004;107(1–2):176–90.

[102] American College of Sports Medicine. American College of Sports Medicine (ACSM) guidelines for exercise testing and prescription. 6th edition. Philadelphia: Lippincot Williams and Wilkins; 2000.

[103] Cohen I, Rainville J. Aggressive exercise as treatment for chronic low back pain. Sports Med 2002;32(1):75–82.

[104] Rainville J, Ahern DK, Phalen L. Altering beliefs about pain and impairment in a functionally oriented treatment program for chronic low back pain. Clin J Pain 1993;9(3): 196–201.

[105] Hayden JA, van Tulder MW, Malmivaara A, et al. Exercise therapy for treatment of nonspecific low back pain. Cochrane Database Syst Rev 2005;3:CD000335.

[106] Van Tulder M, Malmivaara A, Esmail R, et al. Exercise therapy for low back pain: a systematic review within the framework of the Cochrane Collaboration Back Review Group. Spine 2000;25(21):2784–96.

[107] Keller A, Brox JI, Gunderson R, et al. Trunk muscle strength, cross-sectional area, and density in patients with chronic low back pain randomized to lumbar fusion or cognitive intervention and exercises. Spine 2003;29:3–8.

[108] Abenhaim L, Rossignol M, Valat J, et al. The role of activity in the therapeutic management of back pain. Spine 2002;25(4 Suppl):1S–33.

[109] Hurwitz EL, Morgenstern H, Chiao C. Effects of recreational physical activity and back exercises on low back pain and psychological distress: findings from the UCLA Low Back Pain Study. Am J Public Health 2005;95(10):1817–24.

[110] Simons D, Travell J. Myofascial pain and dysfunction: the trigger point manual. 2nd edition. Baltimore (MD): Williams & Wilkins; 1999.

[111] Han SC, Harrison P. Myofascial pain syndrome and trigger-point management. Reg Anesth 1997;22(1):89–101.

[112] Rachlin E. Trigger points. In: Rachlin E, editor. Myofascial pain and fibromyalgia: trigger point management. St. Louis (MO): Mosby; 1994. p. 145–57.

[113] McNulty WH, Gevirtz RN, Hubbard DR, et al. Needle electromyographic evaluation of trigger point response to a psychological stressor. Psychophysiology 1994;31(3):313–6.

[114] Majlesi J, Unalan H. High-power pain threshold ultrasound technique in the treatment of active myofascial trigger points: a randomized, double-blind, case-control study. Arch Phys Med Rehabil 2004;85(5):833–6.

[115] Hou CR, Tsai LC, Cheng KF, et al. Immediate effects of various physical therapeutic modalities on cervical myofascial pain and trigger-point sensitivity. Arch Phys Med Rehabil 2002;83(10):1406–14.

[116] Hong C. Lidocaine injection versus dry needling to myofascial trigger point. The importance of the local twitch response. Am J Phys Med Rehabil 1994;73:256–63.

[117] Porta M. A comparative trial of botulinum toxin type A and methylprednisolone for the treatment of myofascial pain syndrome and pain from chornic muscle spasm. Pain 2000; 85:101–5.

[118] Wheeler A, Goolkasian P, Gretz S. A randomized, double-blind, prospective pilot study of botulinum toxin injection for refractory, unilateral, cervicothoracic, paraspinal, myofascial pain syndrome. Spine 1998;23:1662–6.

[119] Blumenfeld A. Botulinum toxin type A as an effective prophylactic treatment for primary headache disorders. Headache 2003;42:853–60.

[120] Padberg M, De Haan R, Tavy D. Treatment of chronic tension-type headache with botulinum toxin: a double-blind, placebo-controlled clinical trial. Cephalgia 2004;24: 675–80.

[121] Sundaraj R, Ponciano P, Johnstone C, et al. Treatment of chronic refractory intractable headache with botulinum toxin type A: a retrospective study. Pain Pract 2004;4:229–34.

[122] Larsen J. Current considerations in pain management for the patient with fibromylagia syndrome. Pharm Times 1999;66:2HPT–6HPT.

[123] Bradley L, Sotolongo A, Alberts K, et al. Abnormal regional cerebral blood flow in the caudate nucleus among fibromylagia patients and non-patients is associated with insidious symptom onset. J Musculoskeletal Pain 1999;7:285–92.

[124] Russell I, Orr MD, Littman B, et al. Elevated cerebrospinal fluid levels of substance P in patients with the fibromyalgia syndrome. J Bacteriol Virol Immunol [Microbiol] 1994;37: 1593–601.

[125] Bradley L, Weigent D, Sotolongo A, et al. Blood serum levels of nitric oxide (NO) are elevated in women with fibromyalgia (FM): possible contributions to central and peripheral sensitization. Arthrits Rheum 2000;43:S173.

[126] Larson A, Giovengo S, Russell I, et al. Changes in the concentrations of amino acids in the cerebrospinal fluid that correlate with pain in patients with fibromyalgia; implications for nitric oxide pathways. Pain Headache 2000;87:201–11.

[127] Wolfe F, Smythe H, Yunus M, et al. The American College of Rheumatology 1990 criteria for the classification of fibromyalgia: report of the Mutlicenter Criteria Committee. Arthritis Rheum 1990;33:160–72.

[128] Geisser ME, Casey KL, Brucksch CB, et al. Perception of noxious and innocuous heat stimulation among healthy women and women with fibromyalgia: association with mood, somatic focus, and catastrophizing. Pain 2003;102(3):243–50.

[129] Nicassio PM, Radojevic V, Weisman MH, et al. A comparison of behavioral and educational interventions for fibromyalgia. J Rheumatol 1997;24(10):2000–7.

[130] Moldofsky H, Scarisbrick P, England R, et al. Musculosketal symptoms and non-REM sleep disturbance in patients with "fibrositis syndrome" and healthy subjects. Psychosom Med 1975;37(4):341–51.

[131] Goldenberg D, Burchardt C, Crofford L. Management of fibromyalgia syndrome. JAMA 2004;292:2916–22.

[132] Giesecke T, Williams D, Harris R, et al. Subgrouping of fibromyalgia patients on the basis of pressure-pain thresholds and psychological factors. Arthritis Rhuem 2003;48:2916–22.

[133] Carette S, Bell MJ, Reynolds WJ, et al. Comparison of amitriptyline, cyclobenzaprine, and placebo in the treatment of fibromyalgia. A randomized, double-blind clinical trial. Arthritis Rheum 1994;37(1):32–40.

[134] Biasi G, Manca S, Manganelli S, et al. Tramadol in the fibromyalgia syndrome: a controlled clinical trial versus placebo. Int J Clin Pharmacol Res 1998;18(1):13–9.

[135] Arnold LM, Hess EV, Hudson JI, et al. A randomized, placebo-controlled, double-blind, flexible-dose study of fluoxetine in the treatment of women with fibromyalgia. Am J Med 2002;112(3):191–7.

[136] Arnold LM, Lu Y, Crofford LJ, et al. A double-blind, multicenter trial comparing duloxetine with placebo in the treatment of fibromyalgia patients with or without major depressive disorder. Arthritis Rheum 2004;50(9):2974–84.

[137] Sayar K, Aksu G, Ak I, et al. Venlafaxine treatment of fibromyalgia. Ann Pharmacother 2003;37:1561–5.

[138] Valim V, Oliveira L, Suda A, et al. Aerobic fitness effects in fibromyalgia. J Rheumatol 2003;30(5):1060–9.

[139] Gowans S, DeHueck A. Effectiveness of exercise in management of fibromyalgia. Curr Opin Rheumatol 2004;16:138–42.

[140] Jentoft ES, Kvalvik AG, Mengshoel AM. Effects of pool-based and land-based aerobic exercise on women with fibromyalgia/chronic widespread muscle pain. Arthritis Rheum 2001;45(1):42–7.

[141] Rossy LA, Buckelew SP, Dorr N, et al. A meta-analysis of fibromyalgia treatment interventions. Ann Behav Med 1999;21(2):180–91.

[142] Keefe F. Cognitive behavioral therapy for managing pain. Clin Psychol 1996;49:4–5.

[143] Williams D. Psychological and behavioral therapies in fibromyalgia and related syndromes. Best Pract Res Clin Rheum 2003;17:649–65.

[144] Buckelew SP, Conway R, Parker J, et al. Biofeedback/relaxation training and exercise interventions for fibromyalgia: a prospective trial. Arthritis Care Res 1998;11(3):196–209.

[145] Burckhardt C. Multidisciplinary approaches for management of fibromyalgia. Curr Pharm Des 2006;12:59–66.

[146] Pfeiffer A, Thompson J, Nelson A, et al. Effects of a 1.5-day multidisciplinary outpatient treatment program for fibromyalgia: a pilot study. Am J Phys Med Rehabil 2003;82:186–91.

THE MEDICAL
CLINICS
OF NORTH AMERICA

ELSEVIER
SAUNDERS

Med Clin N Am 91 (2007) 97–111

Nonopioid Analgesics

Muhammad A. Munir, MD*, Nasr Enany, MD,
Jun-Ming Zhang, MSc, MD

*Department of Anesthesiology, University of Cincinnati College of Medicine,
231 Albert Sabin Way, PO Box 67031, Cincinnati, OH 45267-0531, USA*

Drug therapy is the mainstay of management for acute, chronic, and cancer pain in all age groups, including neonates, infants, and children. The analgesics include opioids, nonopioid analgesics, and adjuvants or coanalgesics. In this article we will overview various nonopioid analgesics including salicylates, acetaminophen, traditional nonselective nonsteroidal anti-inflammatory drugs (NSAIDs), and cyclooxygenase-2 (COX-2) inhibitors. Unless contraindicated, any analgesic regimen should include a nonopioid drug, even when pain is severe enough to require the addition of an opioid [1].

Nonopioid analgesics

Acetaminophen and NSAIDs are useful for acute and chronic pain resulting from a variety of disease processes including trauma, arthritis, surgery, and cancer [2,3]. NSAIDs are indicated for pain that involves inflammation as an underlying pathologic process because of their ability to suppress production of inflammatory prostaglandins. NSAIDs are both analgesic and anti-inflammatory, and may be useful for the treatment of pain not involving inflammation as well [4].

Nonopioid analgesics differ from opioid analgesics in certain important regards. These differences should be realized to provide the most effective care to acute pain patients and include the following:

1. There is a ceiling effect to the dose response curve of NSAIDs, therefore after achieving an analgesic ceiling, increasing the dose increases the side effects but additional analgesia does not result.

This work was partly supported by Grant No. NS45594 from the National Institutes of Health.

* Corresponding author.
E-mail address: munirma@ucmail.uc.edu (M.A. Munir).

2. NSAIDs don't produce physical or psychological dependence and therefore sudden interruption in treatment doesn't cause drug withdrawals.
3. NSAIDs are antipyretic.

Nonopioid analgesics are underrated for the treatment of chronic pain and unnecessarily omitted for patients with chronic pain and patients unable to take oral medications. Parenteral, topical, and rectal dosage forms are available for some NSAIDs that are often underused.

All NSAIDs, including the subclass of selective COX-2 inhibitors, are anti-inflammatory, analgesic, and antipyretic. NSAIDs are a chemically heterogeneous group of compounds, often chemically unrelated, which nevertheless share certain therapeutic actions and adverse effects. Aspirin also inhibits the COX enzymes but in a manner molecularly distinct from the competitive, reversible, active site inhibitors and is often distinguished from the NSAIDs. Similarly, acetaminophen, which is antipyretic and analgesic but largely devoid of anti-inflammatory activity, also is conventionally segregated from the group despite its sharing NSAID activity with other actions relevant to its clinical action in vivo.

Mechanism of action

All NSAIDs inhibit the enzyme cyclooxygenase (COX), thereby inhibiting prostaglandin synthesis [5]. In addition to peripheral effects, NSAIDs exert a central action at the brain or spinal cord level that could be important for their analgesic effects [6]. More than 30 years ago, multiple isoforms of COX were hypothesized. In 1990s, the second form (COX-2) was isolated. COX-1, the originally identified isoform, is found in platelets, the gastrointestinal (GI) tract, kidneys, and most other human tissues. COX-2 is found predominantly in the kidneys and central nervous system (CNS), and is induced in peripheral tissues by noxious stimuli that cause inflammation and pain. The inhibition of COX-1 is associated with the well-known gastrointestinal bleeding and renal side effects that can occur with NSAID use. The anti-inflammatory therapeutic effects of NSAIDs are largely due to COX-2 and not the COX-1 inhibition. Until recently all available NSAIDs nonselectively inhibited the COX-1 and COX-2 isoforms. Drugs that do so are termed nonselective or traditional NSAIDs. Most NSAIDs inhibit both COX-1 and COX-2 with little selectivity, although some conventionally thought of as nonselective NSAIDs, diclofenac, etodolac, meloxicam, and nimesulide, exhibit selectivity for COX-2 in vitro. Indeed, meloxicam acts as a preferential inhibitor of COX-2 at relatively low doses (eg, 7.5 mg daily).

COX-2 selective NSAIDs that first became available in the late 1990s provide all of the beneficial effects of nonselective NSAIDs but fewer adverse effects on bleeding and the GI tract. COX-2 selective NSAIDs are no safer to the kidneys than nonselective NSAIDs. As of mid-2003, three members of the initial class of COX-2 inhibitors, the coxibs, were approved for use in the United States and Europe. Both rofecoxib and valdecoxib have now been withdrawn from the market in view of their potential cardiovascular adverse event profile. None of the coxibs have established greater clinical efficacy over NSAIDs.

Aspirin covalently modifies COX-1 and COX-2, irreversibly inhibiting cyclooxygenase activity. This is an important distinction from all the NSAIDs because the duration of aspirin's effects is related to the turnover rate of cyclooxygenases in different target tissues. The duration of effect of nonaspirin NSAIDs, which competitively inhibit the active sites of the COX enzymes, relates more directly to the time course of drug disposition. The importance of enzyme turnover in relief from aspirin action is most notable in platelets, which, being anucleate, have a markedly limited capacity for protein synthesis. Thus, the consequences of inhibition of platelet COX-1 last for the lifetime of the platelet. Inhibition of platelet COX-1-dependent thromboxane (TX)A2 formation therefore is cumulative with repeated doses of aspirin (at least as low as 30 mg/day) and takes roughly 8 to 12 days, the platelet turnover time, to recover once therapy has been stopped.

Acetaminophen is a nonsalicylate that may produce similar analgesic and antipyretic potency as aspirin, but has no antiplatelet effects, lacks clinically useful peripheral anti-inflammatory effects, and does not damage the gastric mucosa. A proposed mechanism of acetaminophen is inhibition of a third isoform of cyclooxygenase (COX-3) that was identified recently [7]. COX-3 is only found within the CNS, which would account for the analgesic and antipyretic, but not anti-inflammatory, action of acetaminophen. However, the significance of COX-3 remains uncertain, and the mechanism(s) of action of acetaminophen has yet to be defined.

Clinical uses

All NSAIDs, including selective COX-2 inhibitors, are antipyretic, analgesic, and anti-inflammatory, with the exception of acetaminophen, which is antipyretic and analgesic but is largely devoid of anti-inflammatory activity.

Analgesic

When employed as analgesics, these drugs usually are effective only against pain of low-to-moderate intensity, such as dental pain. Although their maximal efficacy is generally much less than the opioids, NSAIDs lack the unwanted adverse effects of opiates in the CNS, including respiratory depression and the development of physical dependence. NSAIDs do not change the perception of sensory modalities other than pain. Chronic postoperative pain or pain arising from inflammation (eg, somatic pain) is controlled particularly well by NSAIDs.

Antipyretics

NSAIDs reduce fever in most situations, but not the circadian variation in temperature or the rise in response to exercise or increased ambient temperature. It is important to select an NSAID with rapid onset for the management of fever associated with minor illness in adults. Due to the association with Reye's syndrome, aspirin and other salicylates are contraindicated in children and young adults less than 12 years old with fever associated with viral illness.

Anti-inflammatory

NSAIDs have their key application as anti-inflammatory agents in the treatment of musculoskeletal disorders, such as rheumatoid arthritis and osteoarthritis. In general, NSAIDs provide only symptomatic relief from pain and inflammation associated with the disease, and do not arrest the progression of pathological injury to tissue.

Other clinical uses

In addition to analgesic, antipyretic and anti-inflammatory effects, NSAIDs are also used for closure of patent ductus arteriosus in neonates, to treat severe episodes of vasodilatation and hypotension in systemic mastocytosis, treatment of biochemical derangement of Bartter's syndrome, chemoprevention of certain cancers such as colon cancer, and prevention of flushing associated with use of niacin.

Adverse reactions of NSAID treatment

Adverse effects of aspirin and NSAIDs therapy are listed in Table 1 and are considerably common in elderly patients and caution is warranted in choosing an NSAID for pain management in the elderly.

Gastrointestinal

The most common symptoms associated with these drugs are gastrointestinal, including anorexia, nausea, dyspepsia, abdominal pain, and diarrhea. These symptoms may be related to the induction of gastric or intestinal ulcers, which is estimated to occur in 15% to 30% of regular users. The risk is further increased in those with *Helicobacter pylori* infection, heavy alcohol consumption, or other risk factors for mucosal injury, including the concurrent use of glucocorticoids. All of the selective COX-2 inhibitors have been shown to be less prone than equally efficacious doses of traditional NSAIDs to induce endoscopically visualized gastric ulcers [8].

Table 1
Side effects of NSAID therapy

Gastrointestinal	Nausea, anorexia, abdominal pain, ulcers, anemia, gastrointestinal hemorrhage, perforation, diarrhea
Cardiovascular	Hypertension, decreased effectiveness of anti-hypertensive medications, myocardial infarction, stroke, and thromboembolic events (last three with selective COX-2 inhibitors); inhibit platelet activation, propensity for bruising and hemorrhage
Renal	Salt and water retention, edema, deterioration of kidney function, decreased effectiveness of diuretic medication, decreased urate excretion, hyperkalemia, analgesic nephropathy
Central nervous system	Headache, dizziness, vertigo, confusion, depression, lowering of seizure threshold, hyperventilation (salicylates)
Hypersensitivity	Vasomotor rhinitis, asthma, urticaria, flushing, hypotension, shock

Gastric damage by NSAIDs can be brought about by at least two distinct mechanisms. Inhibition of COX-1 in gastric epithelial cells depresses mucosal cytoprotective prostaglandins, especially PGI_2 and PGE_2. These eicosanoids inhibit acid secretion by the stomach, enhance mucosal blood flow, and promote the secretion of cytoprotective mucus in the intestine. Another mechanism by which NSAIDs or aspirin may cause ulceration is by local irritation from contact of orally administered drug with the gastric mucosa.

Co-administration of the PGE_1 analog, misoprostol, or proton pump inhibitors (PPIs) in conjunction with NSAIDs can be beneficial in the prevention of duodenal and gastric ulceration [9].

Cardiovascular

Selective inhibitors of COX-2 depress PGI_2 formation by endothelial cells without concomitant inhibition of platelet thromboxane. Experiments in mice suggest that PGI_2 restrains the cardiovascular effects of TXA_2, affording a mechanism by which selective inhibitors might increase the risk of thrombosis [10,11]. This mechanism should pertain to individuals otherwise at risk of thrombosis, such as those with rheumatoid arthritis, as the relative risk of myocardial infarction is increased in these patients compared with patients with osteoarthritis or no arthritis. The incidence of myocardial infarction and stroke has diverged in such at-risk patients when COX-2 inhibitors are compared with traditional NSAIDs [12]. Placebo-controlled trials have now revealed that there may be an increased incidence of myocardial infarction and stroke in patients treated with rofecoxib [13], valdecoxib [14], and celecoxib [15], suggesting potential for a mechanism-based cardiovascular hazard for the class, ie, selective COX-2 inhibitors (although not equal for all agents) [16].

Blood pressure, renal, and renovascular adverse events

Traditional NSAIDs and COX-2 inhibitors have been associated with renal and renovascular adverse events [17]. NSAIDs have little effect on renal function or blood pressure in normal human subjects. However, in patients with congestive heart failure, hepatic cirrhosis, chronic kidney disease, hypovolemia, and other states of activation of the sympathoadrenal or renin-angiotensin systems, prostaglandin formation and effects in renal blood flow/renal function becomes significant in both model systems and in humans [18].

Analgesic nephropathy

Analgesic nephropathy is a condition of slowly progressive renal failure, decreased concentrating capacity of the renal tubule, and sterile pyuria. Risk factors are the chronic use of high doses of combinations of NSAIDs and frequent urinary tract infections. If recognized early, discontinuation of NSAIDs permits recovery of renal function.

Hypersensitivity

Certain individuals display hypersensitivity to aspirin and NSAIDs, as manifested by symptoms that range from vasomotor rhinitis with profuse watery secretions, angioedema, generalized urticaria, and bronchial asthma to laryngeal edema, bronchoconstriction, flushing, hypotension, and shock. Aspirin intolerance is a contraindication to therapy with any other NSAID because cross-sensitivity can provoke a life-threatening reaction reminiscent of anaphylactic shock. Despite the resemblance to anaphylaxis, this reaction does not appear to be immunological in nature.

Although less common in children, this syndrome may occur in 10% to 25% of patients with asthma, nasal polyps, or chronic urticaria, and in 1% of apparently healthy individuals.

Pharmacokinetics and pharmacodynamics

Most of the NSAIDs are rapidly and completely absorbed from the gastrointestinal tract, with peak concentrations occurring within 1 to 4 hours. Aspirin begins to acetylate platelets within minutes of reaching the presystemic circulation. The presence of food tends to delay absorption without affecting peak concentration. Most NSAIDs are extensively protein-bound (95% to 99%) and undergo hepatic metabolism and renal excretion. In general, NSAIDs are not recommended in the setting of advanced hepatic or renal disease due to their adverse pharmacodynamic effects (Tables 2 and 3).

Selected nonopioid analgesics: clinical pearls

Salicylates

Salicylates include acetylated aspirin (acetylsalicylic acid) and the modified salicylate diflunisal, which is a diflurophenyl derivative of salicylic acid. Aspirin was invented in 1897; it is one of the oldest nonopioid oral analgesics. Gastric disturbances and bleeding are common adverse effects with therapeutic doses of aspirin. Because of the possible association with Reye's syndrome, aspirin should not be used for children younger than the age of 12 with viral illness, particularly influenza.

Salicylate salts (nonacetylated)

Salicylate salts such as choline magnesium trisalicylate and salsalate are effective analgesics and produce fewer GI side effects than aspirin [19]. Unlike aspirin and other nonselective NSAIDs, therapeutic doses do not greatly affect bleeding time or platelet aggregation tests in patients without prior clotting abnormalities [20].

Acetaminophen

Acetaminophen is a nonsalicylate that may produce similar analgesic and antipyretic potency as aspirin, but has no antiplatelet effects, lacks clinically useful peripheral anti-inflammatory effects, and does not damage the gastric mucosa. Although acetaminophen is well tolerated at recommended doses of up to 4000 mg/day, acute overdoses can cause potentially fatal hepatic necrosis. Patients with chronic alcoholism and liver disease and patients who are fasting can develop severe hepatotoxicity, even at usual therapeutic doses [21]. The Food and Drug Administration (FDA) now requires alcohol warnings for acetaminophen as well as all other nonprescription analgesics [22]. Acetaminophen overdoses are common because acetaminophen is a frequent ingredient in many nonprescription and prescription analgesic formulations. Acetaminophen has a reduced risk of ulcers and ulcer complications when compared with nonselective NSAIDs and is rarely associated with renal toxicity. Acetaminophen is an underrecognized cause of over-anticoagulation with warfarin in the outpatient setting [23].

Pyrrolacetic acids

Ketorolac is a pyrrolacetic acid, which is available in injection form. An initial dose of 30 mg followed by 10 to 15 mg intravenously (IV) every 6 hours is equianalgesic to 6 to 12 mg of IV morphine. Ketorolac may precipitate renal failure especially in elderly and hypovolemic patients. It is therefore recommended to limit use of Ketorolac to 5 days only. Also, clinicians should try to use the lowest dose felt to be needed.

Table 2
Nonopioid analgesics: comparative pharmacology

Drug	Proprietary names (not all-inclusive)	Average oral analgesic dose, mg	Dose interval, h	Maximal daily dose, mg	Analgesic efficacy compared to standards	Plasma half-life, h	Comments
Acetaminophen	Numerous	500–1,000	4–6	4000	Comparable to aspirin	2–3	Rectal suppository available for children and adults. Sustained-release preparation available, >2g/day may increase INR in patients receiving Warfarin.
Salicylates	Numerous	500–1000	4–6	4000		0.25	Because of risk of Reye's syndrome, do not use in children under 12 with possible viral illness. Rectal suppository available for children and adults. Sustained-release preparation available.
Acetylated Aspirin							

Modified							
Diflunisal	Dolobid	1000 initial, 500 subsequent	8–12	1500	500 mg superior to aspirin 650 mg, with slower onset and longer duration; an initial dose of 1000 mg significantly shortens time to onset	8–12	Dose in elderly 500–1000 mg/day — Does not yield salicylate
Salicylate salts							
Choline magnesium trisalicylate	Trilisate	1000–1500	12	2000–3000	Longer duration of action than aspirin 650 mg	9–17	Unlike aspirin and NSAIDs, does not increase bleeding time
	Tricosal						
NSAIDs							
Propionic acids							
Ibuprofen	Motrin, Rufen, Nuprin, Advil, Medipren, others	200–400	4–6	2400	Superior at 200 mg to aspirin 650 mg	2–2.5	Most commonly used NSAID in US. Available without prescription.
Naproxen	Naprosyn	500 initial, 250 subsequent	6–8	1500	—	12–15	Better tolerated than indomethacin and aspirin.
	Naprolan						

(continued on next page)

Table 2 (*continued*)

Drug	Proprietary names (not all-inclusive)	Average oral analgesic dose, mg	Dose interval, h	Maximal daily dose, mg	Analgesic efficacy compared to standards	Plasma half-life, h	Comments
Naproxen sodium	Anaprox	550 initial, 275 subsequent	6–8	1650	275 mg comparable to aspirin, 650 mg, with slower onset and longer duration; 550 mg superior to aspirin 650 mg		
Naproxen sodium	Aleve	220 mg	8–12	—	Comparable to aspirin	2–3	—
Fenoprofen	Nalfon	200	4–6	3200	Superior at 25 mg to aspirin 650 mg	1.5	Sustained-release preparation available
Ketoprofen	Orudis	25–50	6–8	300			
Ketoprofen OTC	Actron, Orudis-K+	12.5–25	4–6	—			
Oxaprozin	Daypro	600	12–24	1200		24–69	
Indolacetic acids							
Indomethacin	Indocin Indocin, SR Indochron E-R				Comparable to aspirin 650 mg	2	Not routinely used because of high incidence of gastrointestinal and Central nervous system side effects; rectal and sustained-release oral forms available for adults

Phenylacetic acid

Diclofenac potassium has been shown to be superior in efficacy and analgesic duration to aspirin and also inhibits selectively more COX-2 then COX-1.

Enolic acids

Meloxicam has long half-life and roughly 10-fold COX-2 selectivity on average in ex vivo assays [24]. There is significantly less gastric injury compared with piroxicam (20 mg/d) in subjects treated with 7.5 mg/d of meloxicam, but the advantage is lost with 15 mg/d [25].

Naphthylalkanone

Nabumetone is a prodrug; it is absorbed rapidly and is converted in the liver to one or more active metabolites, principally 6-methoxy-2-naphtylacetic acid, a potent nonselective inhibitor of COX [26]. The incidence of gastrointestinal ulceration appears to be lower than with other NSAIDs [27] (perhaps because of its being a prodrug or the fact that there is essentially no enterohepatic circulation).

Propionic acids

Ibuprofen and naproxen are the most commonly used NSAIDs in the United States. These are available without a prescription in the United States. The relative risk of myocardial infarction appears unaltered by ibuprofen, but it is reduced by around 10% with naproxen, compared with a reduction of 20% to 25% by aspirin. Ibuprofen and naproxen are better tolerated than aspirin and indomethacin and have been used in patients with a history of gastrointestinal intolerance to other NSAIDs.

Indolacetic acids

Indomethacin is a more potent inhibitor of the cyclooxygenase than is aspirin, but patient intolerance generally limits its use to short-term dosing. A very high percentage (35% to 50%) of patients receiving usual therapeutic doses of indomethacin experience untoward symptoms. CNS side effects, indeed the most common side effects, include severe frontal headache, dizziness, vertigo, and light-headedness; mental confusion and seizure may also occur, severe depression, psychosis, hallucinations, and suicide have also been reported. Caution must be exercised when starting indomethacin in elderly patients, or patients with history of epilepsy, psychiatric disorders, or Parkinson's disease, because they are greater risk of CNS adverse effects.

COX-2 selective inhibitors

Three members of the initial class of COX-2 inhibitors, the coxibs, were approved for use in the United States. Both rofecoxib and valdecoxib have now been withdrawn from the market in view of their adverse event profile.

Table 3
Selected nonopioid analgesics: analgesic dosage and comparative efficacy to standards

Drug	Proprietary names (not all-inclusive)	Average oral analgesic dose, mg	Dose interval, h	Maximal daily dose, mg	Analgesic efficacy compared to standards	Plasma half-life, h	Comments
Sulindac	Clinoril	150	12	400		7.8 Activemeta = 16	
Etodolac	Lodine	300–400	8–12	1000	More potent than sulindac and naproxen, but less potent than indomethacin		
Pyrrolacetic acids							
Ketorolac	Toradol	30 or 60 mg IM or 30 mg IV initial, 15 or 30 mg IV or IM subsequent	6	150 first day, 120 thereafter	In the range of 6–12 mg of morphine	6	Limit treatment to 5 days; may precipitate renal faiure in dehydrated patients, average dose in elderly 10–15 mg IM/IV Q6 h
Tolmetin	Tolectin	200–600	8	1800		5	
Anthranilic acids							
Mefenamic acid	Ponstel	500 initial, 250 subsequent	6	1500	Comparable to aspirin 650 mg	2	In US use is restricted to interval of 1 week

Phenylacetic acids							
Diclofenac potassium	Cataflam	50 mg	8	150	Superior in efficacy and analgesic duration to aspirin 650 mg		More selective for COX-2 than COX-1
Enolic acids							
Meloxicam	Mobic	7.5–15	24	15		15–20	Ten-fold selective for COX-2
Piroxicam	Feldene	20–40	24	40		50	
Naphthylalkanone							
Nabumetone	Relafen	1000 initial 500–750 subsequent	8–12	2000	Pain relief equal to aspirin, indomethacin, naproxen, and sulindac	24	Fewer gastrointestinal side effects
Cox-2 selective							
Celecoxib	Celebrex	200–400	12–24	400	Anti-inflammatory and analgesic effect similar to naproxen	11	
Rofecoxib	Vioxx	12.5–50	24	25		17	
Valdecoxib	Bextra	10–20	12–24	50 up to 5 days 40		8–11	

Valdecoxib has been associated with a threefold increase in cardiovascular risk in two studies of patients undergoing cardiovascular bypass graft surgery [28]. Based on interim analysis of data from the Adenomatous Polyp Prevention on Vioxx (APPROVe) study, which showed a significant (twofold) increase in the incidence of serious thromboembolic events in subjects receiving 25 mg of rofecoxib relative to placebo [13], rofecoxib was withdrawn from the market worldwide [29]. The FDA advisory panel agreed that rofecoxib increased the risk of myocardial infarction and stroke and that the evidence accumulated was more substantial than for valdecoxib and appeared more convincing than for celecoxib. Effects attributed to inhibition of prostaglandin production in the kidney (hypertension and edema) may occur with nonselective COX inhibitors and also with celecoxib. Studies in mice and some epidemiological evidence suggest that the likelihood of hypertension on NSAIDs reflects the degree of inhibition of COX-2 and the selectivity with which it is attained. Thus, the risk of thrombosis, hypertension, and accelerated atherogenesis may be mechanistically integrated. The coxibs should be avoided in patients prone to cardiovascular or cerebrovascular disease. None of the coxibs has established clinical efficacy over NSAIDs. While selective COX-2 inhibitors do not interact to prevent the antiplatelet effect of aspirin, it now is thought that they may lose some of their gastrointestinal advantage over NSAIDs alone when used in conjunction with aspirin.

Summary

NSAIDs are useful analgesics for many pain states, especially those involving inflammation. Their use is frequently overlooked in patients with postoperative and chronic pain. Unless there is a contraindication, the use of an NSAID should be routinely considered to manage acute pain, chronic cancer, and noncancer pain.

References

[1] Acute Pain Management Guideline Panel. Acute pain management: operative or medical procedures and trauma: clinical practice guidelines. Rockville (MD): Agency for Healthcare Policy and Research, Public Health Service, US Department of Health and Human Services; 1992.
[2] Carr D, Goudas L. Acute pain. Lancet 1999;353:2051–8.
[3] Zuckerman L, Ferrante F. Nonopioid and opioid analgesics. In: Ashburn M, Rice L, editors. The management of pain. Philadelphia (PA): Churchill-Livingstone; 1998. p. 111–40.
[4] McCormack K. Non-steroidal anti-inflammatory drugs and spinal nociceptive processing. Pain 1994;59:9–43.
[5] Vane J. Inhibition of prostaglandin synthesis as a mechanism of action for aspirin-like drugs. Nature 1971;234:231–8.
[6] Malmberg A, Yaksh T. Hyperalgesia mediated by spinal glutamate or substance P receptor blocked by spinal cyclooxygenase inhibition. Science 1992;257:1276–9.
[7] Chandrasekharan N, Dai H, Roos K, et al. COX-3, a cyclooxygenase-1 variant inhibited by acetaminophen and other analgesic/antipyretic drugs: cloning, structure, and expression. Proc Natl Acad Sci U S A 2002;99:13926–31.

[8] Deeks JJ, Smith LA, Bradley MD. Efficacy, tolerability, and upper gastrointestinal safety of celecoxib for treatment of osteoarthritis and rheumatoid arthritis: systematic review of randomised controlled trials. BMJ 2002;325:619–26.

[9] Rostom A, Dube C, Wells G, et al. Prevention of NSAID-induced gastroduodenal ulcers. Cochrane Database Syst Rev 2002;4:CD002296.

[10] McAdam BF, Catella-Lawson F, Mardini IA, et al. Systemic biosynthesis of prostacyclin by cyclooxygenase (cox)-2: the human pharmacology of a selective inhibitor of COX-2. Proc Natl Acad Sci U S A 1999;96:272–7.

[11] Catella-Lawson F, McAdam B, Morrison BW, et al. Effects of specific inhibition of cyclooxygenase-2 on sodium balance, hemodynamics, and vasoactive eicosanoids. J Pharmacol Exp Ther 1999;289:735–41.

[12] FitzGerald GA. COX-2 and beyond: approaches to prostaglandin inhibition in human disease. Nat Rev Drug Discov 2003;2:879–90.

[13] Bresalier RS, Sandler RS, Quan H, et al. Cardiovascular events associated with rofecoxib in a colorectal adenoma chemoprevention trial. N Engl J Med 2005;352:1092–102.

[14] Nussmeier NA, Whelton AA, Brown MT, et al. Complications of COX-2 inhibitors parecoxib and valdecoxib after cardiac surgery. N Engl J Med 2005;352:1081–91.

[15] Solomon SD, McMurray JV, Pfeffer MA, et al. Cardiovascular risk associated with celecoxib in a clinical trial for colorectal adenoma prevention. N Engl J Med 2005;352:1071–80.

[16] Pitt B, Pepine C, Willerson JT. Cyclooxygenase-2 inhibition and cardiovascular events. Circulation 2002;106:167–9.

[17] Cheng HF, Harris RC. Cyclooxygenases, the kidney, and hypertension. Hypertension 2004; 43:525–30.

[18] Patrono C, Dunn MJ. The clinical significance of inhibition of renal prostaglandin synthesis. Kidney Int 1987;32:1–12.

[19] Ehrlich G. Primary drug therapy: aspirin vs. the nonsteroidal anti-inflammatory drugs. Postgrad Med 1983;May Spec:9–17.

[20] Stuart JJ, Pisko EJ. Choline magnesium trisalicylate does not impair platelet aggregation. Pharmatherapeutica 1981;2(8):547–51.

[21] Whitcomb D, Block G. Association of acetaminophen hepatotoxicity with fasting and ethanol use. JAMA 1994;272:1845–50.

[22] Food and Drug Administration. Over-the-counter drug products containing analgesic/antipyretic active ingredients for internal use; required alcohol warning; final rule; compliance date. Food and Drug Administration, HHS, Fed Regist 1999;64(51):13066–7.

[23] Hylek E, Heiman H, Skates S, et al. Acetaminophen and other risk factors for excessive warfarin anticoagulation. JAMA 1998;279:657–62.

[24] Panara MR, Renda G, Sciulli MG, et al. Dose-dependent inhibition of platelet cyclooxygenase-1 and monocyte cyclooxygenase-2 by meloxicam in healthy subjects. J Pharmacol Exp Ther 1999;290:276–80.

[25] Patoia L, Santucci L, Furno P, et al. A 4-week, double-blind, parallel-group study to compare the gastrointestinal effects of meloxicam 7.5 mg, meloxicam 15 mg, piroxicam 20 mg and placebo by means of faecal blood loss, endoscopy and symptom evaluation in healthy volunteers. B Brit J Rheumatol 1996;35:61–7.

[26] Patrignani P, Panara MR, Greco A, et al. Biochemical and pharmacological characterization of the cyclooxygenase activity of human blood prostaglandin endoperoxide synthases. J Pharmacol Exp Ther 1994;271:1705–12.

[27] Scott DL, Palmer RH. Safety and efficacy of nabumetone in osteoarthritis: emphasis on gastrointestinal safety. Aliment Pharmacol Ther 2000;14:443–52.

[28] Furberg CD, Psaty BM, FitzGerald GA. Parecoxib, valdecoxib and cardiovascular risk. Circulation 2005;111:249.

[29] FitzGerald GA. Coxibs and cardiovascular disease. N Engl J Med 2004;351:1709–11.

THE MEDICAL
CLINICS
OF NORTH AMERICA

Med Clin N Am 91 (2007) 113–124

Adjuvant Analgesics

Helena Knotkova, PhD[a],*, Marco Pappagallo, MD[b]

[a]Department of Pain Medicine and Palliative Care, 353 E 17th Street, Gilman Hall, Unit 4C,
Beth Israel Medical Center, New York, NY 10003, USA
[b]Department of Anesthesiology, Mount-Sinai Hospital, One Gustave L. Levy Place,
1190 Fifth Avenue, New York, NY 10029, USA

Adjuvant analgesics are a diverse group of drugs that were originally developed for a primary indication other than pain. Many of these medications are currently used to enhance analgesia under specific circumstances [1]. Of interest, a few of these agents are currently used as primary analgesics for specific pain conditions as well as adjuvants in some other pain conditions.

The proper use of adjuvant drugs is one of the keys to success in effective pain management. Since adjuvant analgesics are typically administered to patients who take multiple medications, decisions regarding administration and dosage must be made with a clear understanding of the stage of the disease and the goals of care [2,3]. Since adjuvants cause their own side effects, they are better be used when a patient cannot obtain satisfactory pain relief from a primary pain medication (ie, acetaminophen, nonsteroidal anti-inflammatory drugs, opioids). As a general recommendation, adjuvants should not be used only to lower the opioid dose in functional patients whose pain is well controlled with minimum side effects.

Antidepressants

Antidepressants play an important role in the treatment of chronic pain, as they display a wide variety of interactions with the neuraxis nociceptive pathways: monoamine modulation, opioid interactions, descending inhibition, and ion-channel blocking [4,5]. Tricyclic antidepressants (TCAs), such as amitriptyline, nortriptyline, and desipramine, inhibit both serotonin and norepinephrine reuptake to varying degrees, and are effective for most

There is no funding related to this chapter.
* Corresponding author.
E-mail address: HKnotkov@chpnet.org (H. Knotkova).

neuropathic conditions [5]. The use of TCAs should be closely monitored for relatively frequent, poorly tolerated adverse effects, including cardiotoxicity, confusion, urinary retention, orthostatic hypotension, nightmares, weight gain, drowsiness, dry mouth, and constipation.

Serotonin and noradrenaline reuptake inhibitors (SNRIs), eg, duloxetine and venlafaxine lack the anticholinergic and antihistamine effects of the TCAs [6–8]. Venlafaxine has been shown to modulate allodynia and pinprick hyperalgesia in human experimental models and to relieve neuropathic pain in breast cancer, perhaps by broadening its monoamine coverage by inhibiting the presynaptic uptake of both serotonin, norepinephrine, and, to a lesser extent, dopamine. Duloxetine has recently been approved by the Food and Drug Administration (FDA) for the treatment of pain secondary to diabetic neuropathy. Another antidepressant, *bupropion*, which inhibits the reuptake of dopamine, has also shown evidence to be effective for the treatment of neuropathic pain [9].

Selective serotonin reuptake inhibitors (SSRIs), such as paroxetine and fluoxetine, are effective antidepressants, but relatively ineffective analgesics. While being used for the management of comorbidities such as anxiety, depression, and insomnia, which frequently affect patients with chronic neuropathic pain, SSRIs have not shown the same efficacy as the TCAs in the treatment of neuropathic pain [10].

Anticonvulsants

Antiepileptic drugs (AEDs) are becoming the most promising agents for the management of neuropathic pain, given their propensity to dampen neuronal excitability. These qualities have made some AEDs first-line treatment in neuropathic conditions. The application of AEDs for pain stems from the shared pathophysiology of neuropathic pain and epilepsy. Neuronal hyperexcitability characterizes both conditions. The hyperexcitable state of neuropathic pain is characterized by reduced thresholds (sensitization) and ectopic discharges at the spinal dorsal horn or dorsal root ganglion (DRG) pain-signaling neurons due to, for example, the up-regulation of Na^+ and Ca^{++} membrane channels [11].

The gabapentinoid AEDs, gabapentin and pregabalin, have both established efficacy for neuropathic pain. Gabapentin and pregabalin act on neither gamma-aminobutyric acid (GABA) receptors nor sodium channels. In fact, they modulate cellular calcium influx into nociceptive neurons by binding to voltage-gated calcium channels, in particular to the alpha-2-delta subunit of the channel [12,13]. Gabapentin has been regarded as the first-line treatment for neuropathic pain syndromes, likely because of its favorable toxicity profile and lack of major drug interactions [14,15]. Therefore, when used specifically for neuropathic pain, gabapentinoid AEDs should be considered primary analgesics and not adjuvants any longer [15–18]. In a recent randomized, double-blind, active placebo-controlled, crossover trial [19], patients with neuropathic pain received either active placebo (lorazepam) or controlled-release morphine, gabapentin, and a combination of gabapentin and morphine, each treatment given orally for 5 weeks. The study indicated that the best analgesia was obtained from the gabapentin/morphine combination, with each medication given at a lower dose than when given as a single agent [19]. Additionally, other studies [20–22] have demonstrated that the concomitant administration of gabapentin reduces opioid requirements in the postoperative setting [20,21]. Side effects of gabapentin tend to occur early in treatment. The most common adverse events include somnolence, dizziness, ataxia, fatigue, impaired concentration, and edema. Pregabalin is also known to cause weight gain.

Another AED, carbamazepine, is very effective in the treatment of trigeminal neuralgia (a neuropathic condition characterized by brief excruciating lancinating pains), however the side effects and the need to monitor hematologic function are significant drawbacks that have often persuaded physicians to use other drugs, especially oxcarbamazepine, which is the keto-analog of carbamazepine. Oxcarbamazepine binds to sodium channels in their inactive state, increases potassium channel conductance, and modulates high-voltage activated calcium channels [23]. Oxcarbamazepine has been used at times successfully in the treatment of neuropathic pain syndromes. The most commonly observed adverse events are dizziness, somnolence, diplopia, fatigue, nausea, abnormal vision, and hyponatremia. Thus, Na^+ level should be monitored.

Lamotrigine has shown some efficacy for carbamazepine-resistant trigeminal neuralgia [24]. The benefit of lamotrigine may be from its blocking tetrodotoxin-resistant Na^+ channels [25] and from an inhibition of glutamate release from presynaptic neurons [26]. Lamotrigine has been widely studied in both animals and humans with some evidence pointing toward effectiveness in pain control. Preliminary observations and study have suggested the potential usefulness of lamotrigine for pain associated with diabetic neuropathy, multiple sclerosis, spinal cord injury, central poststroke pain, polyneuropathy, complex regional pain syndrome, and trigeminal neuralgia [27–30].

Several new AEDs, eg, levetiracetam, zonisamide, and tiagabine, along with topiramate, may have analgesic effect in primary headaches [13,30]. Topiramate has also been used anecdotally in the treatment of complex regional pain syndrome (CRPS) type 1 [31].

Alpha-2-adrenergic agonists

Alpha-2 adrenergic agonists are known to have a spinal antinociceptive effect via alpha-2 receptor subtypes [32]. Clonidine, a well-known alpha-2 adrenergic agonist, produces a synergistic antinociceptive effect with opioids

[33]. In addition to being a primary analgesic when given intrathecally in the postoperative period, clonidine potentiates the analgesic benefit of opioids [34].

Tizanidine is a relatively short-acting, oral alpha-2 adrenergic agonist with a much lower hypotensive effect than clonidine. Tizanidine has been mostly used for the management of spasticity. However, animal studies and clinical experience indicate some usefulness of tizanidine for a variety of painful states, including neuropathic pain disorders [35–37].

Corticosteroids

Corticosteroids, eg, prednisone and dexamethasone, are effective as adjuvants for patients with inflammatory neuropathic pain from peripheral nerve injuries. In addition, corticosteroids have been used successfully to treat bone pain, pain from bowel obstruction, pain from lymphedema, and headache pain associated with intracranial pressure. Analgesic effect has been described for prednisone and dexamethasone in a broad range of doses. However, no analgesic studies have been performed about the relative potency among corticosteroids, long-term efficacy, and dose-response relationship. Short-term use of high doses of steroids is mainly recommended for patients whose pain rapidly escalates with functional impairment. The risk of adverse events increases with the dose and with the duration of therapy, and involves edema, dyspeptic symptoms, candidiasis, and occasional gastrointestinal bleeding.

Local anesthetics

The local anesthetics operate on the principle of decreasing neuronal excitability at the level of Na^+ channels that propagate action potentials. This channel blockade has an effect on both spontaneous pain and evoked pain [38]. An interesting point about these analgesic properties is that they occur at subanesthetic doses—lidocaine suppresses the frequency rather than the duration of Na^+ channel opening [39,40]. In addition, animal models suggest that both topical and central anesthetics may exhibit synergism with morphine [41,42].

Transdermal lidocaine shows a good efficacy for postherpetic pain [43]. In a controlled clinical trial, the transdermal form of 5% lidocaine relieved pain associated with post herpetic neuralgia (PHN) without significant adverse effects [44]. There are also observations that suggest some benefit for other neuropathic pain states [45], including diabetic neuropathy [46], CRPS, postmastectomy pain, and HIV-related neuropathy [47]. Intravenous lidocaine has also been used in patients with neuropathic pain [48].

The anti-arrhythmic local anesthetic mexiletine is a sodium channel blocker with analgesic properties for neuropathic pain similar to those of some AEDs (eg, lamotrigine, carbamazepine). Mexiletine is contraindicated in the presence of second- and third-degree atrium-ventricular conduction blocks. In addition, the incidence of gastrointestinal side effects (eg, diarrhea, nausea) is quite high in patients taking mexiletine.

Topical agents

A typical topical agent is capsaicin. Capsaicin, the natural substance in hot chili peppers, activates the recently cloned vanilloid neuronal membrane receptor [49,50]. After an initial depolarization, a single administration of a large dose of capsaicin appears to produce a prolonged deactivation of capsaicin-sensitive nociceptors [51,52]. The analgesic effect is dose-dependent and may last for several weeks. Studies at low capsaicin concentrations (0.075% or less) have shown mixed results, possibly a result of noncompliance. At the present time, preparations of injectable capsaicin and local anesthetics are being developed for site-specific, moderate to severe pain. These preparations should provide pain relief in patients with postsurgical, neuropathic, and musculoskeletal pain conditions for weeks or months after a single treatment.

NMDA antagonists

Animal experiments have shown that central and peripheral N-methyl-D-aspartate (NMDA) receptors play an important role in hyperalgesia and chronic pain [53]. NMDA antagonists dextromethorphan, methadone, memantine, amantadine, and ketamine seem to be effective in the management of hyperalgesic neuropathic states poorly responsive to opioid analgesics [53]. Ketamine when used as an adjuvant to opioids appears to increase pain relief by 20% to 30% and allows opioid dose reduction by 25% to 50% [54,55]. However, ketamine has a narrow therapeutic window and can cause intolerable side effects, such as hallucinations and memory impairment.

Of interest is the possibility that NMDA antagonists, such as D-methadone, memantine, and dextromethorphan, may prevent or counteract opioid analgesic tolerance [56,57].

Cannabinoids

Delta(9)-trans-tetrahydrocannabinol (Δ-9-THC) is the most widely studied cannabinoid. Evidence from animal studies and clinical observations indicate that cannabinoids have some analgesic properties [56,58,59]. Analgesic sites of action have been identified in brain areas, in the spinal cord, and in the periphery. Cannabinoids appear to have a peripheral anti-inflammatory action, and induce antinociception at lower doses than those obtained from effective central nervous system (CNS) concentrations.

In contrast to the strong preclinical data, good clinical evidence on the efficacy of cannabinoids is lacking. CNS depression seems to be the predominant limiting adverse effect. In chronic neuropathic pain, $1'$, $1'$-dimethyl-heptyl-Δ8-tetrahydrocannabinol-11-oic acid (CT-3), a THC-11-oic acid analog, at a dose of 40 mg/d, has shown to be more effective than placebo and to produce no major unfavorable side effects [59].

Interestingly, the addition of inactive doses of cannabinoids to low doses of opioid mu agonists appears to potentiate opioid antinociception. Moreover, cannabinoids appear to have a predominant anti-allodynic/antihyperalgesic effect [56,58–60].

Bisphosphonates and calcitonin

Bisphosphonate therapy has proven highly valuable in the management of numerous bone-related conditions, including hypercalcemia, osteoporosis, multiple myeloma, and Paget's disease. Bisphosphonates, synthetic analogs of pyrophosphate, bind with a high affinity to the bone hydroxyapatite crystals and reduce bone resorption by inhibiting osteoclastic activity. Earlier bisphosphonates, such as etidronate, have been largely replaced by the use of second-generation bisphosphonates, including pamidronate, as well as third-generation bisphosphonates, including zolendronic acid and ibandronate. Multiple studies have demonstrated the efficacy of second- and third-generation bisphosphonates in pain reduction for bone metastases [61–64]. Zolendronic acid and ibandronate provide significant and sustained relief from metastatic bone pain, improving patient functioning and quality of life.

Bisphosphonates have been reported to be efficacious not only in bone cancer pain, but also in the treatment of CRPS, a neuropathic inflammatory pain syndrome [65,66]. However, the underlying mechanism of bisphosphonate analgesic effect is poorly understood. It may be related to the inhibition and apoptosis of activated phagocytic cells such as osteoclasts and macrophages. This leads to a decreased release of proinflammatory cytokines in the area of inflammation. In animal models of neuropathic pain (sciatic nerve ligature), bisphosphonates reduced the number of activated macrophages infiltrating the injured nerve, reduced Wallerian nerve fiber degeneration, and decreased experimental hyperalgesia [67]. One adverse event that has recently emerged in a number of oncology patients treated with the most potent bisphosphonates is osteonecrosis of the jaw. The disorder affects patients with cancer on bisphosphonate treatment for multiple myeloma or bone metastasis from breast, prostate, or lung cancer. Risk factors include prolong duration of bisphosphonate treatment (ie, monthly intravenous administration for more than 1 to 2 years), poor oral hygiene, and a history of recent dental extraction.

Calcitonin may have several pain-related indications in patients who have bone pain, including osseous metastases. The most frequent routes of absorption are intranasal and subcutaneous injection. Calcitonin reduces resorption of bone by inhibiting osteoclastic activity and osteolysis [68].

GABA agonists

Baclofen is an analog of the inhibitory neurotransmitter gamma-amino-butyric acid (GABA) and has a specific action on the GABA-B receptors. It has been used for many years as an effective spasmolytic agent. Baclofen also has shown anecdotal evidence of effectiveness in the treatment of tri-geminal neuralgia [69]. Clinical experience supports the use of low-dose ba-clofen to potentiate the antineuralgic effect of carbamazepine for trigeminal neuralgia. Baclofen also has been used intrathecally to relieve intractable spasticity, and it may have a role as an adjuvant when added to spinal opi-oids for the treatment of intractable neuropathic pain and spasticity. The most common side effects of baclofen are drowsiness, weakness, hypoten-sion, and confusion. It is important to note that discontinuation of baclofen always requires a slow tapering to avoid the occurrence of seizures and other severe neurological manifestations.

Neuroimmunomodulatory agents

Several lines of evidence indicate that tumor necrosis factor (TNF)-alpha, as well as other proinflammatory interleukins, may play a key role in the mechanism of inflammatory neuropathic pain. Neutralizing antibodies to TNF-alpha and interleukin-1 receptor may become an important therapeu-tic approach for severe inflammatory pain resistant to nonsteroidal anti-inflammatory drugs (NSAIDs), as well as for certain forms of neuropathic inflammatory pain [70–72]. Thalidomide has been shown to prevent hyper-algesia caused by nerve constriction injury in rats [73,74] and thalidomide is known to inhibit TNF-alpha production. TNF-alpha antagonists or newly developed thalidomide analogs with a better safety profile may play a rele-vant role in the prevention and treatment of otherwise intractable painful disorders [75]. Finally, inhibitors of microglia activation and of the tran-scription factor known as NF-κB are being explored and these lines of research may open new exciting treatment avenues.

Summary

Chronic pain, whether arising from viscera, bone, or any other tissue or structure, is, more often than commonly thought, the result of a mixture of pain mechanisms, and therefore there is no simple formula available to manage chronic complex pain states. Box 1 summarizes a pharmacological

---

Box 1. Analgesic algorithm for difficult-to-treat pain syndromes

Pharmacological Interventions[1]
Moderate to severe pain/functional impairment; pain with a score
of > 4 on the on the brief pain inventory [76]

1. Gabapentinoid (gabapentin, pregabalin) ± Opioid/opioid
   rotation **or**
2. *Antidepressant* (TCA, duloxetine, venlafaxine) ± *Opioid/opioid*
   rotation **or**
3. *Gabapentinoid + antidepressant + Opioid/opioid rotation*; in
   addition, may consider trials of one or more of the following
   adjuvants when clinically appropriate:

   > *Topical therapies* for cutaneous allodynia/hyperalgesia[2]
   > *Anti-inflammatory drugs* (corticosteroids for acute
   >   inflammatory neuropathic pain)
   > *IV bisphosphonates* for cancer bone pain or CRPS/RSD
   > *Non-gabapentinoid AEDs* such as carbamazepine or
   >   oxcarbazepine or lamotrigine ± baclofen for intermittent
   >   lancinating pain due to cranial neuralgias
   > *NMDA antagonists*
   > *Mexiletine*

   ---

   [1] On a compassionate basis, according to the patient's clinical condition and
   pain mechanism, the physician may want to consider an empirical trial of one
   or more of the emergent topical, oral or parenteral/intrathecal therapies as
   discussed in the text.
   [2] If SMP, consider topical clonidine and sympatholytic interventions; if
   clinically feasible, trials of topical therapies, eg, lidocaine 5% patch, may be
   considered for a variety of pain states and features.

---

algorithm for difficult-to-treat chronic pain, which merely introduces the
medication aspect of the treatment. In effect, any comprehensive algorithm
should call for an interdisciplinary approach that would include rehabilitation, as well as psychosocial, and when indicated, interventional techniques.

The major rationale for introducing adjuvants is to better balance efficacy
and adverse effects. The following scenarios should prompt the use of adjuvants in clinical practice:

- The toxic limit of a primary analgesic has been reached.
- The therapeutic benefit of a primary analgesic has plateaued, eg, treatment has reached its true efficacy limit or pharmachodynamic tolerance
  has developed.
- The primary analgesic is contraindicated, eg, substance abuse, aberrant
  behavior, organ failure, allergy, and so forth.

- Subjective and qualitative symptoms demand broader coverage. Patients often convey that different medications will impart distinct analgesic benefits.
- Presence of disabling nonpainful complaints and need to manage symptoms such as insomnia, depression, anxiety, and fatigue that all cause worsening of the patient's quality of life and function.

Physicians have also been drawn to the adjuvants secondary to new realities of clinical practice. Moreover, aversion to addiction and diversion remains a potent force that shapes prescribing profiles.

References

[1] Wallenstein DJ, Portenoy RK. Nonopioid and adjuvant analgesics. In: Berger AM, Portenoy RK, Weissman DE, editors. Principles and practice of palliative care and supportive oncology. New York: Lippincott; 2002. p. 435–55.
[2] Banning A, Sjogren P, Henriksen H. Pain causes in 200 patients referred to a multidisciplinary cancer pain clinic. Pain 1991;45:45–8.
[3] Black DR, Sang CN. Advances and limitations in the evaluation of analgesic combination therapy. Neurology 2005;65(12, Suppl 4):S3–6.
[4] Sindrup SH, Otto M, Finnerup NB, et al. Antidepressants in the treatment of neuropathic pain. Basic Clin Pharmacol Toxicol 2005;96(6):399–409.
[5] Saarto T, Wiffen PJ. Antidepressants for neuropathic pain. Cochrane Database Syst Rev 2005;3:CD005454.
[6] Marchand F, Alloui A, Pelissier T, et al. Evidence for an antihyperalgesic effect of venlafaxine in vincristine-induced neuropathy in rat. Brain Res 2003;980:117–20.
[7] Grothe DR, Scheckner B, Albano D. Treatment of pain syndromes with venlafaxine. Pharmacotherapy 2004;24:621–9.
[8] Rowbotham MC, Goli V, Kunz NR, et al. Venlafaxine extended release in the treatment of painful diabetic neuropathy: a double-blind, placebo-controlled study. Pain 2004;110:697–706.
[9] Semenchuk MR, Sherman S, Davis B. Double-blind, randomized trial of bupropion SR for the treatment of neuropathic pain. Neurology 2001;57:1583–8.
[10] Max MB, Lynch SA, Muir J, et al. Effects of desipramine, amitriptyline, and fluoxetine on pain in diabetic neuropathy. N Engl J Med 1992;326:1250–6.
[11] Han HC, Lee DH, Chung JM. Characteristics of ectopic discharges in a rat neuropathic pain model. Pain 2000;84(2–3):253–61.
[12] Matthews EA, Dickenson AH. Effects of spinally delivered N- and P-type voltage-dependent calcium channel antagonists on dorsal horn neuronal responses in a rat model of neuropathy. Pain 2001;92:235–46.
[13] Shi W, Liu H, Zhang Y, et al. Design, synthesis, and preliminary evaluation of gabapentin-pregabalin mutual prodrugs in relieving neuropathic pain. Arch Pharm (Weinheim) 2005; 338:358–64.
[14] Bennett M, Simpson K. Gabapentin in the treatment of neuropathic pain. Palliat Med 2004; 18:5–11.
[15] Rowbotham M, Harden N, Stacey B, et al. Gabapentin for the treatment of postherpetic neuralgia: a randomized controlled trial. JAMA 1998;280:1837–42.
[16] Backonja M, Beydoun A, Edwards KR, et al. Gabapentin for the symptomatic treatment of painful neuropathy in patients with diabetes mellitus: a randomized controlled trial. JAMA 1998;280:1831–6.
[17] Rice AS, Maton S. Gabapentin in postherpetic neuralgia: a randomized, double blind, placebo-controlled study. Pain 2001;94:215–24.

[18] Wiffen P, Collins S, McQuay H, et al. Anticonvulsant drugs for acute and chronic pain [systematic review]. Cochrane Pain, Palliative and Supportive Care Group. Cochrane Database Syst Rev 2005;4:CD.

[19] Gilron I, Bailey JM, Tu D, et al. Morphine, gabapentin, or their combination for neuropathic pain. N Engl J Med 2005;352:1324–34.

[20] Eckhardt K, Ammon S, Hofmann U, et al. Gabapentin enhances the analgesic effect of morphine in healthy volunteers. Anesth Analg 2000;91(1):185–91.

[21] Turan A, Karamanlioglu B, Memis D, et al. Analgesic effects of gabapentin after spinal surgery. Anesthesiology 2004;100(4):935–8.

[22] Tallarida RJ. Drug synergism: its detection and applications. J Pharmacol Exp Ther 2001; 298(3):865–72.

[23] Ichikawa K, Koyama N. Inhibitory effect of oxacarbamazepine on high-frequency firing in peripheral nerve fibers. Eur J Pharmacol 2001;42:119–22.

[24] Zakrzewska JM, Chaudhry Z, Nurmikko TJ, et al. Lamotrigine (lamictal) in refractory trigeminal neuralgia: results from a double-blind, placebo controlled, crossover trial. Pain 1997;73:223–30.

[25] Brau ME, Dreimann M, Olschewski A, et al. Effect of drugs used for neuropathic pain management on tetrodotoxin-resistant NaC currents in rat sensory neurones. Anesthesiology 2001;94:137–44.

[26] McNamara J. Drugs acting on the central nervous system. In: Harman G, Limbird LE, Morinoff PB, et al, editors. Goodman and Gilman's the pharmacological basis of therapeutics. 9th edition. New York: McGraw-Hill; 1996. p. 461–86.

[27] Vestergaard K, Andersen G. Lamotrigine for central poststroke pain: a randomized controlled trial. Neurology 2001;56:184–90.

[28] Webb J, Kamali F. Analgesic effect of lamotrigine and phenytoin on cold-induced pain: a cross-over placebo conrolled study in healthy volunteers. Pain 1998;76:357–63.

[29] Steiner TJ, Findley LJ, Yuen AW. Lamotrigine versus placebo in the prophylaxis of migraine with and without aura. Cephalgia 1997;17:109–12.

[30] Pappagallo M. Newer antiepileptic drugs: possible uses in the treatment of neuropathic pain and migraine. Clin Ther 2003;25:2506–38.

[31] Pappagallo M. Preliminary experience with topiramate in the treatment of chronic pain syndromes. Presented at the 17th Annual Meeting of the American Pain Society, San Diego, 1998.

[32] Khasar SG, Green PG, Chou B, et al. Peripheral nociceptive effects of alpha 2-adrenergic receptor agonists in the rat. Neuroscience 1995;66(2):427–32.

[33] Yaksh Tl, Malmberg AB. Pharmacological approaches to the treatment of chronic pain: new concepts and critical issues. Progress in pain research and management. Vol 1. Interaction of spinal modulatory receptor systems. Seattle: IASP Press; 1994. p. 151–71.

[34] Goudas LC, Carr DB, Filos KS, et al. The spinal clonidine-opioid analgesic interaction: from laboratory animals to the postoperative ward. A review of preclinical and clinical evidence. Analgesia 1998;3:277–90.

[35] Fogelholm R, Murros K. Tizanidine in chronic tension-type headache: a placebo controlled double-blind cross-over study. Headache 1992;32:509–13.

[36] Fromm GH, Aumentado D, Terrence CF. A clinical and experimental investigation of the effects of tizanidine in trigeminal neuralgia. Pain 1993;53:265–71.

[37] Semenchuk MR, Sherman S. Effectiveness of tizanidine in neuropathic pain: an open-label study. J Pain 2000;1(4):285–92.

[38] Cummins TR, Waxman SG. Downregulation of tetrodotoxin-resistant sodium currents and upregulation of a rapidly repriming tetrodotoxin-sensitive sodium current in small spinal sensory neurons after nerve injury. J Neurosci 1997;17(10):3503–14.

[39] Rowbotham MC, Reisner-Keller LA, Fields HL. Both intravenous lidocaine and morphine reduce the pain of postherpetic neuralgia. Neurology 1991;41(7):1024–8.

[40] Lai J, Hunter JC, Porreca F. The role of voltage-gated sodium channels in neuropathic pain. Curr Opin Neurobiol 2003;13:291–7.

[41] Saito Y, Kaneko M, Kirihara Y, et al. Interaction of intrathecally infused morphine and lidocaine in rats (part I): synergistic antinociceptive effects. Anesthesiology 1998;89: 1455–63.
[42] Kolesnikov YA, Chereshnev I, Pasternak GW. Analgesic synergy between topical lidocaine and topical opioids. J Pharmacol Exp Ther 2000;295(2):546–51.
[43] Galer BS, Rowbotham MC, Perander J, et al. Topical lidocaine patch relieves postherpetic neuralgia more effectively than a vehicle topical patch: results of an enriched enrollment study. Pain 1999;80:533–8.
[44] Rowbotham MC, Davies PS, Verkempinck C, et al. Lidocaine patch: double-blind controlled study of a new treatment method for post-herpetic neuralgia. Pain 1996;65:39–44.
[45] Devers A, Galer BS. Topical lidocaine patch relieves a variety of neuropathic pain conditions: an open-label study. Clin J Pain 2000;16:205–8.
[46] Hart-Gouleau S, Gammaitoni A, Galer B, et al. Open label study of the effectiveness and safety of lidocaine patch 5% (Lidoderm) in patients with painful diabetic neuropathy [abstract]. Pain Medicine 2005;6:379–84.
[47] Berman SM, Justis JV, HO M, et al. Lidocaine patch 5% (Lidoderm) significantly improves quality of life (QOL) in HIV-associated painful periperal neuropathy [abstract 205]. In: Program and abstracts of the IASP 10th World Congress of Pain. Seattle: IASP, 2002.
[48] Wallace MS. Calcium and sodium channel antagonists for the treatment of pain. Clin J Pain 2000;16:S80–5.
[49] Caterina MJ, Schumacher MA, Tominaga M, et al. The capsaicin receptor: a heat-activated ion channel in the pain pathway. Nature 1997;389:816–24.
[50] Knotkova H, Pappagallo M. Pharmacology of pain transmission and modulation: peripheral mechanisms. In: Pappagallo M, editor. The neurological basis of pain. New York: McGraw-Hill; 2005. p. 53–61.
[51] Robbins WR, Staats PS, Levine J, et al. Treatment of intractable pain with topical large-dose capsaicin: preliminary report. Anesth Analg 1998;86:579–83.
[52] Vyklicky L, Knotkova H, Vitaskova Z, et al. Inflammatory mediators at acidic pH activate capsaicin receptor in cultured sensory neurons from newborn rats. J Neurophysiol 1998;79: 670–6.
[53] Bennett GJ. Update on the neurophysiology of pain transmission and modulation: focus on the NMDA-receptor. J Pain Symptom Manage 2000;9:S2–6.
[54] Fitzgibbon EJ, Viola R. Parenteral ketamine as an analgesic adjuvant for severe pain: development and retrospective audit of a protocol for a palliative care unit. J Palliat Med 2005;8: 49–57.
[55] Lossignol DA, Obiols-Portis M, Body JJ. Successful use of ketamine for intractable cancer pain. Support Care Cancer 2005;13:188–93.
[56] Davis AM, Inturrisi CE. d-Methadone blocks morphine tolerance and N-methyl-D-aspartate-induced hyperalgesia. J Pharmacol Exp Ther 1999;289:1048–53.
[57] Price DD, Mayer DJ, Mao J, et al. NMDA-receptor antagonists and opioid receptor interactions as related to analgesia and tolerance. J Pain Symptom Manage 2000;19:S7–11.
[58] Richardson JD. Cannabinoids modulate pain by multiple mechanisms of action. J Pain 2000; 1(1):2.
[59] Karst M, Salim K, Burstein S, et al. Analgesic effect of the synthetic cannabinoid CT-3 on chronic neuropathic pain: a randomized controlled trial. JAMA 2003;290:1757–62.
[60] Richardson JD, Aanonsen L, Hargreaves KM. Antihyperalgesic effects of spinal cannabinoids. Eur J Pharmacol 1998;345(2):145–53.
[61] Smith MR. Osteoclast-targeted therapy for prostate cancer. Curr Treat Options Oncol 2004; 5:367–75.
[62] Mystakidou K, Katsouda E, Stathopoulou E, et al. Approaches to managing bone metastases from breast cancer: the role of bisphosphonates. Cancer Treat Rev 2005;31:303–11.
[63] Wardley A, Davidson N, Barrett-Lee P, et al. Zoledronic acid significantly improves pain scores and quality of life in breast cancer patients with bone metastases: a randomized,

crossover study of community vs hospital bisphosphonate administration. Br J Cancer 2005; 92:1869–76.

[64] Lerner UH. Neuropeptidergic regulation of bone resorption and bone formation. J Musculoskelet Neuronal Interact 2002;2:440–7.

[65] Cortet B, Flipo RM, Coquerelle P, et al. Treatment of severe, recalcitrant reflex sympathetic dystrophy: assessment of efficacy and safety of the second generation bisphosphonate pamidronate. Clin Rheumatol 1997;16:51–6.

[66] Varenna M, Zucchi F, Ghiringhelli D, et al. Intravenous clodronate in the treatment of reflex sympathetic dystrophy syndrome. A randomized, double blind, placebo controlled study. J Rheumatol 2000;27:1477–83.

[67] Liu T, van Rooijen N, Tracey DJ. Depletion of macrophages reduces axonal degeneration and hyperalgesia following nerve injury. Pain 2000;86:25–32.

[68] Szanto J, Ady N, Jozsef S. Pain killing with calcitonin nasal spray in patients with malignant tumors. Oncology 1992;49:180–2.

[69] Sindrup SH, Jensen TS. Pharmacotherapy of trigeminal neuralgia. Clin J Pain 2002;18(1): 22–7.

[70] Schafers M, Brinkhoff J, Neukirchen S, et al. Combined epineurial therapy with neutralizing antibodies to tumor necrosis factor-alpha and interleukin-1 receptor has an additive effect in reducing neuropathic pain in mice. Neurosci Lett 2001;310:113–6.

[71] Pedersen LH, Nielsen AN, Blackburn-Munro G. Anti-nociception is selectively enhanced by parallel inhibition of multiple subtypes of monoamine transporters in rat models of persistent and neuropathic pain. Psychopharmacology (Berl) 2005;182(4):551–61.

[72] Sevcik MA, Ghilardi JR, Peters CM, et al. Anti-NGF therapy profoundly reduces bone cancer pain and the accompanying increase in markers of peripheral and central sensitization. Pain 2005;115:128–41.

[73] Sommer C, Marziniak M, Myers RR. The effect of thalidomide treatment on vascular pathology and hyperalgesia caused by chronic constriction injury of rat nerve. Pain 1998;74: 83–91.

[74] Ribeiro RA, Vale ML, Ferreira SH, et al. Analgesic effect of thalidomide on inflammatory pain. Eur J Pharmacol 2000;391:97–103.

[75] George A, Marziniak M, Schafers M, et al. Thalidomide treatment in chronic constrictive neuropathy decreases endoneurial tumor necrosis factor-alpha, increases interleukin-10 and has long-term effects on spinal cord dorsal horn met-enkephalin. Pain 2000;88:267–75.

[76] Cleeland CS, Salek S. Compendium of QL instruments. Brief pain inventory. Chichester (West Sussex): Wiley; 1998. p. 1–5.

ELSEVIER
SAUNDERS

THE MEDICAL
CLINICS
OF NORTH AMERICA

Med Clin N Am 91 (2007) 125–139

Topical Analgesics

Gary McCleane, MD

Rampark Pain Centre, 2 Rampark Dromore Road, Lurgan BT66 7JH, Northern Ireland, UK

Among the drugs with well-known peripheral effects are nonsteroidal anti-inflammatory drugs (NSAIDs), local anesthetics, and capsaicin. Less well appreciated is the fact that nitrates, tricyclic antidepressants (TCAs), glutamate receptor antagonists, α-adrenoerecptor antagonists, and cannabinoids may have an analgesic effect when applied topically. The rational for the analgesic effects of these compounds, when applied topically, is discussed in this article.

To patients, it makes sense to apply pain relief directly to where they feel pain. They "know" that oral medication can produce side effects, whereas topical agents are less likely to do so. Knowledgeable physicians, however, understand that pain is influenced by peripheral and central factors. They understand that significant opportunity exists to augment inhibitory or to lessen facilitatory influences on the pain stimulus, and therefore, in general, seem to prefer systemically active agents. Increasing evidence, however, backed up by clinical use, now suggests that topically applied medication can be at least as effective as that administered by the oral route and, in general, has a more favorable side effect profile than orally active agents. In this article, the author looks at medications that have a tradition of topical use and at newer additions to this range of drugs. Although a rich variety of potential pharmacologic targets exists peripherally, to date, only some of these are amenable to currently available therapeutic entities; it is on these that concentration is focused.

Not all medication applied to the skin has a local, peripheral action. Drugs such as fentanyl and buprenorphine, which can be applied to the skin, have predominately central effects. This type of administration is known as "transdermal" to distinguish it from the "topical" analgesics—drugs that are applied to skin and have a predominate peripheral effect.

E-mail address: gary@mccleane.freeserve.co.uk

Anti-inflammatory agents

Nonsteroidal anti-inflammatory drugs

Among the most widely used topical agents are the NSAIDs. These agents are known to reduce the production of prostaglandins that sensitize nerve endings at the site of injury. This effect occurs due to the inhibition of the cyclooxygenase (COX) enzyme that converts arachidonic acid liberated from the phospholipid membrane by phospholipases to prostanoids such as prostaglandin. At least two forms of COX are thought to be important. COX1 is normally expressed in tissues such as stomach and kidneys and plays a physiologic role in maintaining tissue integrity [1]. A second form, COX2, plays a role in pain and inflammation [1]. The analgesic effects of NSAIDs can be dissociated from anti-inflammatory effects, and this may reflect additional spinal and supraspinal actions of NSAIDs to inhibit various aspects of central pain processing [2]. Recent evidence suggests that a third COX, COX3, which is predominately centrally distributed, may also be involved in NSAID or acetaminophen action [3]; however, its role remains uncertain.

When NSAIDs are applied topically, bioavailability and plasma concentrations are 5% to 15% of those achieved by systemic delivery [4]. In human experimental pain models, topically applied NSAIDs produce analgesia in models of cutaneous pain [5–8] and muscle pain [9]. In terms of clinical use, three major reviews—one examining use in musculoskeletal and soft tissue pain [10], another looking at data accrued in over 10,000 patients in 86 trials [11], and the last looking primarily at chronic rheumatic disease [4]—concluded that there was clear and significant evidence that topical NSAIDs have pain-relieving properties.

When NSAIDs are applied topically, relatively high concentrations occur in the dermis, whereas levels in adjacent muscle are as high as when the NSAID is given systemically [4]. Gastrointestinal side effects occur less frequently than when the drug is given orally but are still more likely in patients who have previously demonstrated such responses to oral medication [10].

Perhaps the greatest danger of topical NSAID use is the risk of polypharmacy. A number of over-the-counter topical and oral NSAIDs are now available, and the risk of overdosing with several different preparations taken at the same time and all containing NSAID is very real.

Nitrates

Conventionally used in the treatment of ischemic heart disease, it now seems that nitrates also have potent analgesic and anti-inflammatory effects. It is known that exogenous nitrates stimulate the release of nitric oxide (NO) [12]. This substance is known to be a potent mediator in a wide variety of different cellular systems such as the endothelium and the central and peripheral nervous system. It is released from the endothelium and from neutrophils and macrophages—all known to be intimately involved in the inflammatory process. It appears that NO exerts its effect by stimulating increases in guanylate cyclase, thereby increasing levels of 3′,5′-cyclic GMP [13]. Cholinergic drugs such as acetylcholine produce analgesia in a similar fashion by releasing NO and increasing NO at the nociceptor level [14].

In addition to this action, NO may activate ATP-sensitive potassium channels and activate peripheral antinociception [15]. Endogenous NO levels may be increased if glutamate levels are increased [16]. Glutamate is known to be an excitatory amino acid, activating N-methyl-D-aspartate (NMDA) receptors, thereby initiating sensitization and protracting the pain process.

Topical nitrate, in the form of glyceryl trinitrate (GTN), has been shown to effectively reduce the pain of osteoarthritis [17], supraspinatus tendonitis [18], and infusion-related thrombophlebitis [19]. In addition, it may reduce the pain and inflammation caused by sclerosant treatment of varicose veins [20] and may even be useful in the treatment of vulvar pain [21]. A number of reports suggest that topical nitrates may enhance the analgesic effectiveness of strong opioids [22–24], but it is likely that this effect is due to systemic absorption of the nitrate and a consequent central action. The predominant side effect associated with topical nitrate use is headache. Currently, patch formulations deliver a relatively large amount of nitrate and, therefore, the incidence of headache is high. Should lower dose patches become available, the utility of this treatment would be increased. GTN is also available in an ointment formulation. Measurement and consistency of dosing are problematic with the ointment formulation, and because there is only a small difference between a potentially analgesic dose and one that causes headache, GTN ointment use is less practical than the use of the patch varieties.

Topical nitrates can therefore be considered when pain is localized and particularly in patients in whom NSAIDs are contraindicated. Nitrates are devoid of the renal, gastrointestinal, and hematologic side effects of NSAIDs.

Local anesthetics

Gels/creams

Several topical local anesthetic preparations are available in gel, cream, and patch form. Amethocaine is available as a gel and lidocaine/prilocaine is presented as a cream. The cream contains a eutectic mixture of lidocaine and prilocaine and its use has become established in the anesthetizing of skin before cannula insertion. It also has demonstrable benefit in reducing the pain of other procedures including lumbar puncture, intramuscular injections, and circumcision [25]. Although lidocaine/prilocaine cream is not

US Food and Drug Administration (FDA) approved for any neuropathic pain condition, several studies have been undertaken in patients who have postherpetic neuralgia (PHN). Two of these studies were uncontrolled and showed a pain-reducing effect [26,27], whereas a randomized controlled study of the same condition failed to show any benefit [28]. Caution should be used with long-term use of this preparation because prilocaine use has been associated with the onset of methemoglobinemia.

Patches

Lidocaine is available in a topically applied patch at a 5% strength. In the United States, this preparation is approved by the FDA for the treatment of PHN. Its efficacy in this pain condition is supported by several trials that also confirm that it is well tolerated [29,30]. Not only can pain levels in patients who have PHN be reduced but measures of quality of life also show improvement [31]. In one study of patients who had PHN, 66% of subjects reported reduced pain intensity when up to three lidocaine 5% patches were used for 12 hours each day [31].

Although lidocaine 5% is indicated for use in PHN, it may also be efficacious in other pain conditions. When used in the treatment of focal neuropathic pain conditions such as mononeuropathies and intercostal and ilioinguinal neuralgia, one controlled study confirmed a pain-reducing effect [32]. In an open-label study of 16 patients who had "refractory" neuropathic pain (including patients who had post-thoracotomy pain, complex regional pain syndrome, postamputation pain, neuroma pain, painful diabetic neuropathy, meralgia parasthetica, and postmastectomy pain), 81% of subjects experienced notable pain relief [33]. In this report, *refractory* was defined as those who had failed to gain pain relief or who experienced unacceptable side effects with opiates, anticonvulsants, antidepressants, or antiarrhythmic agents.

Capsaicin

Capsaicin use has a long history in medical practice. Extract of chili pepper was reported in the midnineteenth century to reduce chilblain pain and toothache [34]. It has now been shown to reduce the pain associated with painful diabetic neuropathy [35–38], PHN [39–41], chronic distal painful polyneuropathy [42], oral neuropathic pain [43], surgical neuropathic pain [44], and the pain associated with Guillain-Barré syndrome [45]. In the treatment of non-neuropathic pain, capsaicin has a role, with evidence of a pain-relieving effect in osteoarthritis [46–51] and neck pain [52].

It appears that capsaicin achieves its pain-relieving effect by reversibly depleting sensory nerve endings of substance P [53,54] and by reducing the density of epidermal nerve fibers, also in a reversible fashion [55].

When used clinically, the major impediment to better compliance is the intense burning sensation associated with capsaicin's use. This sensation generally reduces with repeated administration, although when capsaicin cream is applied outside the normal area of application, discomfort is again apparent. It has been shown that coadministration of GTN can reduce the discomfort associated with application [50,56,57] and enhance the analgesic effect of the capsaicin [50]. Alternatively, preapplication of lidocaine 5% cream can also reduce application-associated discomfort [58].

Some patients experience bouts of sneezing when capsaicin is used, which is normally caused by overapplication and drying of the cream on the skin and then nasal inhalation of the capsaicin dust from the application site. Care must always be used so that capsaicin is not applied to moist areas because this is associated with increased burning sensation.

Tricyclic antidepressants

TCAs, when taken orally, have a long pedigree in pain management. Their use is established in a broad range of pain conditions. Their pain-relieving effect is independent of their antidepressant effect. It is unfortunate that their use is also associated with a significant risk of side effects (eg, dry mouth, sedation, urinary retention, and weight gain), which reduces compliance. In contrast, when TCAs are applied topically, side effects are relatively rare, yet a very real chance of pain relief exists. Any relief obtained by topical TCA use can be rationalized by their possible peripheral actions.

Adenosine receptors

At peripheral nerve terminals in rodents, adenosine A_1 receptor activation produces antinociception by decreasing cyclic AMP levels in the sensory nerve terminals, whereas adenosine A_2 receptor activation produces pronociception by increasing cyclic AMP levels in the sensory nerve terminals. Adenosine A_3 receptor activation produces pain behaviors due to the release of histamine and serotonin from mast cells and subsequent actions in the sensory nerve terminal [59]. Caffeine acts as a nonspecific adenosine receptor antagonist. When systemic caffeine is administered with systemic amitriptyline, the normal effect on thermal hyperalgesia is blocked. When amitriptyline is administered into a rodent paw that has neuropathic pain, an antihyperalgesic effect is recorded (but not when it is given into the contralateral paw). This antihyperalgesic effect is blocked by caffeine [60], suggesting that at least part of the effect of peripherally applied amitriptyline is mediated through peripheral adenosine receptors.

Sodium channels

Sudoh and colleagues [61] injected various TCAs by a single injection into rat sciatic notches. These investigators measured the duration of

complete sciatic nerve blockade and compared these values with that of bupivacaine. They found that amitriptyline, doxepin, and imipramine produced a longer complete sciatic nerve block than bupivacaine, whereas
trimipramine and desipramine produced a shorter block. Nortriptyline
and maprotiline failed to produce any block. When the effect of topical application of amitriptyline is compared with that of lidocaine, amitriptyline is
seen to produce longer cutaneous analgesia [62].

These studies suggest, therefore, that from a mode-of-action perspective,
TCAs could have an analgesic effect when applied peripherally.

Animal evidence of an antinociceptive effect of peripherally applied tricyclic antidepressants

Neuropathic pain

When amitriptyline is applied to rodent paws made neuropathic by
a chronic nerve constriction injury, an antinociceptive effect is observed.
When the amitriptyline is applied to the contralateral paw, no antinociceptive effect is observed in the paw on the injured side [63,64]. When desipramine and the selective serotonin reuptake inhibitor fluoxetine are
considered, desipramine has a similar antinociceptive effect when applied
topically, whereas fluoxetine does not [65].

Formalin test

It seems that when amitriptyline [66–68] and desipramine [65] are coad-
ministered peripherally with formalin, the first- and second-phase responses
are reduced.

When amitriptyline is administered peripherally along with formalin, Fos
immunoreactivity in the dorsal region of the spinal cord is significantly
lower than in animals in which formalin is administered alone [68].

Visceral pain

Using a noxious colorectal distension model in the rat, Su and Gebhart
[69] showed that the antidepressants imipramine, desipramine, and clomipr-
amine reduce the response to noxious colorectal distension by 20%, 22%,
and 46%, respectively, compared with control-treated animals.

Thermal injury

Thermal hyperalgesia is produced by exposing a rodent hindpaw to 52°C
for 45 seconds. Locally applied amitriptyline at the time of thermal injury
may produce antihyperalgesic and analgesic effects, depending on the concentration used. When the amitriptyline is applied after the injury, the analgesic effect, but not the antihyperalgesic effect, is retained [70].

Human pain

Human evidence of an analgesic effect with the topical application of
TCAs is limited. A small randomized, placebo-controlled trial of 40 subjects

who had neuropathic pain of mixed etiology produced a reduction of 1.18 on a 0-to-10 linear visual analog score relative to placebo use with the application of a doxepin 5% cream. Minor side effects were seen in only 3 subjects [71]. A larger randomized controlled trial involving 200 subjects, again with neuropathic pain of mixed etiology, suggested that doxepin 5% cream reduced the linear visual analog score by about 1 relative to placebo and that time to effect was about 2 weeks. Again, side effects were minor and infrequent [72]. A pilot study examining the effect of topical amitriptyline application failed to produce any pain relief, but the maximum therapy duration was 7 days [73]; the study may have been terminated before the time to maximal effect had been reached.

Case reports have been made of a useful reduction in pain when doxepin 5% cream was applied topically in subjects who had complex regional pain syndrome type I [74] and when doxepin was used as an oral rinse in patients who had oral pain as a result of cancer or cancer therapy [75].

Although the human evidence of an analgesic effect with topical doxepin is interesting, more study is needed to verify its effects and the effects of other TCAs when used by this route of administration. Evidence suggests that the effect of topically applied doxepin is a local effect and that the consequences of systemic administration and, hence, systemic side effects can be substantially reduced. Doxepin in a 5% cream formulation is currently available and is indicated in the treatment of itch associated with eczema.

Glutamate receptor antagonist

It has recently become apparent that glutamate receptors are expressed on peripheral nerve terminals and that these may contribute to peripheral nociceptive signaling. Ionotropic and metabotropic glutamate receptors are present on membranes of unmyelinated peripheral axons and axon terminals in the skin [76,77], and peripheral inflammation increases the proportions of unmyelinated and myelinated nerves expressing ionotropic glutamate receptors [78]. Local injections of NMDA and non-NMDA glutamate receptor agonists to the rat hindpaw [79,80] or knee joint [81] enhance pain behaviors generating hyperalgesia and allodynia. Injections of metabotropic glutamate receptor agonists produce similar actions [76,82]. Local application of glutamate receptor antagonists inhibits pain behavior following formalin application [81].

In humans, ketamine, a noncompetitive NMDA receptor antagonist, enhances the local anesthetic and analgesic effects of bupivicaine in acute postoperative pain by a peripheral mechanism [83]. When a thermal injury was inflicted in volunteers, one study suggested that subcutaneous injection of ketamine produces long-lasting reduction in hyperalgesia [84], whereas another study failed to confirm this result [85]. That said, not only may any analgesic effect produced by peripheral ketamine application be due to its glutamate receptor activity but ketamine may also block voltage-sensitive calcium channels, alter cholinergic and monoaminergic actions, and interfere with opioid receptors [86–88].

Isolated case reports suggest that topical ketamine can reduce sympathetically maintained pain [89] and pain of malignant origin [90], again suggesting that perhaps glutamate receptor antagonists may have some analgesic effect when applied topically.

α-Adrenoreceptor antagonists

Clonidine, an α_2-adrenoreceptor agonist can be obtained in cream and patch formulations. It can have peripheral and central action when applied topically. Clonidine patches have been reported to reduce the hyperalgesia associated with sympathetically maintained pain but not the hyperalgesia in patients who have sympathetically independent pain [91]. Clonidine cream may also have some pain-relieving effect in orofacial neuralgia-like pain [92]. The effect of clonidine in sympathetically maintained pain may be related to its effect of reducing presynaptic norepinephrine release from sympathetic nerves. In patients who have sympathetically maintained pain, localized norepinephrine injection worsens the mechanical and thermal hyperalgesia in some [93,94] and in those who have peripheral nerve injury [95] and PHN [96].

When clonidine is injected into the knee joint after arthroscopy, pain relief is observed [97,98]; when injected along with bupivicain [99,100] and morphine [101], the analgesic effect of these drugs is enhanced.

Cannabinoids

Cannabinoids (CBs) can act at peripheral sites to produce analgesia by virtue of their effect on CB_1 and CB_2 receptors. In animal models, peripheral administration of agents selective for CB_1 receptors produces local analgesia in the formalin test [102], the carrageenan hyperalgesia model [103], and the nerve injury model [104]. This effect may be obtained because of the effects of these agents on the sensory nerve terminal to inhibit release of calcitonin gene–related peptide [103] or by inhibiting effects of nerve growth factor [105]. CB_2 receptor mechanisms may play a prominent role in inflammatory pain [105].

Opioids

The analgesic effects of systemic opioids are well established and beyond question. Recently, transdermal formulations of fentanyl and buprenorphine have been introduced. Although they are applied to skin, it is likely that their predominant effect is central.

It is now apparent that opioid receptors are not exclusively located in the central nervous system. It appears that opioid receptors are synthesized in dorsal root ganglia and transported into peripheral terminals of primary afferent neurons [106,107]. Both mu and delta opioid receptors can be identified in fine cutaneous nerves in opioid-naïve animals [108]. When a ligature is placed on the rat sciatic nerve, β-endorphin binding sites accumulate proximally and distally to the ligature site [109]. When inflammation is induced, the number of β-endorphin binding sites on both sides of the ligature massively increases [109].

From the human clinical perspective, a number of reports suggest that the knowledge of a peripheral representation of opioid receptors may have practical application. Topical morphine, provided as an oral rinse, has been shown to reduce mucositis-related pain in patients undergoing chemotherapy for head and neck carcinomas [110,111], whereas other case reports suggest that topical opioids may reduce pain from skin ulcer [112,113]. In patients undergoing dental extractions, mixed results have been obtained, with some reporting enhanced relief when morphine is applied locally after dental extraction [114,115] and others reporting no such effect [116]. It has also been suggested that intravesical, strong opioids can reduce painful bladder spasms [117,118].

Despite these suggestions from the literature, two systematic reviews failed to find any evidence of a pain-relieving effect when morphine was used by peripheral application [119,120].

Summary

Our knowledge and understanding of the pathophysiology and treatment of pain is increasing; however, we should not lose sight of the simple opportunities that exist for intercepting pain at peripheral targets. Although systemic medication often has peripheral and central modes of action, the appeal for provision of medication close to where these peripheral targets exist should be high. If these sites can be attacked with relatively high concentrations of active drug while keeping systemic levels of that drug below the level at which systemic side effects become apparent, then this should lead to desirable outcomes. Even though the number of true topical agents with an indication for this use is small, a number of other topical agents are available that evidence suggests have the possibility of being effective. Given the increased understanding of pain, the likelihood of further topical agents becoming available is high.

References

[1] Vane JR, Bakhle YS, Botting J. Cyclo-oxygenase 1 and 2. Annu Rev Pharmacol Toxicol 1998;38:97–120.

[2] Yaksh TL, Dirig DM, Malmberg AB. Mechanisms of action of nonsteroidal anti-inflammatory drugs. Cancer Investig 1998;16:509–27.

[3] Chandrasekharan NV, Dai H, Roos KL, et al. Cox-3, a cyclo-oxygenase-1 variant inhibited by acetaminophen and other analgesic/antipyretic drugs. Cloning, structure and expression. Proc Natl Acad Sci U S A 2002;99:13926–31.

[4] Heyneman CA, Lawless-Liday C, Wall GC. Oral versus topical NSAIDs in rheumatic diseases. A comparison. Drugs 2000;60:555–74.

[5] Kress M, Reeh PW. Chemical excitation and sensitization in nociceptors. In: Cavero F, Belmonte C, editors. Neurobiology and nociceptors. Oxford (UK): Oxford University Press; 1996. p. 258–97.

[6] Steen KH, Reeh PW, Kreysel HW. Topical acetylsalicylic, salicylic acid and indomethacin suppresses pain from experimental tissue acidosis in human skin. Pain 1995;62:339–47.

[7] Steen KH, Reeh PW, Kreysel HW. Dose-dependent competitive block by topical acetylsalicylic acid and salicylic acid of low pH-induced cutaneous pain. Pain 2001;64:71–82.

[8] Schmelz M, Kress M. Topical acetylsalicylate attenuates capsaicin induced pain, flare and allodynia but not thermal hyperalgesia. Neurosci Lett 1996;214:72–4.

[9] Steen KH, Wegner H, Meller ST. Analgesic profile of peroral and topical ketoprofen upon low pH-induced muscle pain. Pain 2001;93:23–33.

[10] Vaile JH, Davis P. Topical NSAIDs for musculoskeletal conditions. A review of the literature. Drugs 1998;56:783–99.

[11] Moore RA, Tramer MR, Carrol D, et al. Quantitative systematic review of topically applied non-steroidal anti-inflammatory drugs. BMJ 1998;316:333–8.

[12] Feelisch M, Noack EA. Correlation between nitric oxide formation during degradation of organic nitrates and activation of guanylate cyclase. Eur J Pharmacol 1987;139:19–30.

[13] Knowles RG, Palacios M, Palmer RM, et al. Formation of nitric oxide from L-arginine in the central nervous system: a transduction mechanism for stimulation of soluble guanylate cyclase. Proc Natl Acad Sci U S A 1989;86:5159–62.

[14] Duarte ID, Lorenzetti BB, Ferreira SH. Acetylcholine induces peripheral analgesia by the release of nitric oxide. In: Moncada S, Higgs A, editors. Nitric oxide from L-arginine. A bioregulatory system. Amsterdam: Elsevier; 1990. p. 165–70.

[15] Soares A, Leite R, Patsuo M, et al. Activation of ATP sensitive K channels: mechanisms of peripheral antinociceptive action of the nitric oxide donor, sodium nitroprusside. Eur J Pharmacol 2000;14:67–71.

[16] Okuda K, Sakurada C, Takahashi M, et al. Characterization of nociceptive responses and spinal release of nitric oxide metabolites and glutamate evoked by different concentrations of formalin in rats. Pain 2001;92:107–15.

[17] McCleane GJ. The addition of piroxicam to topically applied glyceryl trinitrate enhances its analgesic effect in musculoskeletal pain: a randomised, double-blind, placebo-controlled study. Pain Clin 2000;12:113–6.

[18] Berrazueta JR, Losada A, Poveda J, et al. Successful treatment of shoulder pain syndrome due to supraspinatus tendonitis with transdermal nitroglycerin. A double blind study. Pain 1996;66:63–7.

[19] Berrazeuta JR, Poveda JJ, Ochoteco JA, et al. The anti-inflammatory and analgesic action of transdermal glyceryl trinitrate in the treatment of infusion related thrombophlebitis. Postgrad Med J 1993;69:37–40.

[20] Berrazueta JR, Fleitas M, Salas E, et al. Local transdermal glyceryl trinitrate has an anti-inflammatory action on thrombophlebitis induced by sclerosis of leg varicose veins. Angiology 1994;45:347–51.

[21] Walsh KE, Berman JR, Berman LA, et al. Safety and efficacy of topical nitroglycerin for treatment of vulvar pain in women with vulvodynia: a pilot study. J Gend Specif Med 2002;5:21–7.

[22] Lauretti GR, de Oliveira R, Reis MP, et al. Transdermal nitroglycerine enhances spinal sufentanil postoperative analgesia following orthopaedic surgery. Anesthesiology 1999;90: 734–9.

[23] Lauretti GR, Lima IC, Reis MP. Oral ketamine and transdermal nitroglycerin as analgesic adjuvants to oral morphine therapy for cancer pain management. Anesthesiology 1999;90: 1528–33.

[24] Lauretti GR, Perez MV, Reis MP, et al. Double-blind evaluation of transdermal nitroglycerine as an adjuvant to oral morphine for cancer pain management. J Clin Anesth 2002;14: 83–6.

[25] Galer BS. Topical medications. In: Loeser JD, editor. Bonica's management of pain. Philadelphia: Lippincott-Williams & Wilkins; 2001. p. 1736–41.

[26] Attal N, Brasseur L, Chauvin M. Effects of single and repeated applications of a eutectic mixture of local anesthetics (EMLA®) cream on spontaneous and evoked pain in postherpetic neuralgia. Pain 1999;81:203–9.

[27] Litman SJ, Vitkun SA, Poppers PJ. Use of EMLA® cream in the treatment of post-herpetic neuralgia. J Clin Anesth 1996;8:54–7.

[28] Lycka BA, Watson CP, Nevin K, et al. EMLA® cream for the treatment of pain caused by post-herpetic neuralgia: a double-blind, placebo controlled study. Proceedings of the Annual Meeting of the American Pain Society. Glenview (IL): American Pain Society; 1996. A111 (abstract).

[29] Rowbotham MC, Davies PS, Verkempinck C, et al. Lidocaine patch: double-blind controlled study of a new treatment method for post-herpetic neuralgia. Pain 1996;65:39–44.

[30] Galer BS, Rowbotham MC, Perander J, et al. Topical lidocaine patch relieves post-herpetic neuralgia more effectively than vehicle patch: results of an enriched enrolment study. Pain 1999;80:533–8.

[31] Katz NP, Davis MW, Dworkin RH. Topical lidocaine patch produces a significant improvement in mean pain scores and pain relief in treated PHN patients: results of a multi-center open-label trial. J Pain 2001;2:9–18.

[32] Meier T, Wasner G, Faust M, et al. Efficacy of lidocaine 5% patch in treatment of focal peripheral neuropathic pain syndromes: a randomized, double-blind, placebo-controlled study. Pain 2003;106:151–8.

[33] Devers A, Galer BS. Topical lidocaine patch relieves a variety of neuropathic pain conditions: an open-label study. Clin J Pain 2000;16:205–8.

[34] Capsaicin Study Group. Treatment of painful diabetic neuropathy with topical capsaicin. Arch Intern Med 1991;151:2225–9.

[35] Tandan R, Lewis GA, Krusinski PB, et al. Topical capsaicin in painful diabetic neuropathy. Diabetes Care 1992;15:8–13.

[36] Capsaicin Study Group. Effect of treatment with capsaicin on daily activities of patients with painful diabetic neuropathy. Diabetes Care 1992;15:159–65.

[37] Chad DA, Aronin N, Lundstorm R, et al. Does capsaicin relieve the pain of diabetic neuropathy? Pain 1990;42:387–8.

[38] Bernstein JE, Korman NJ, Bickers DR, et al. Topical capsaicin treatment of chronic postherpetic neuralgia. J Am Acad Dermatol 1989;21:265–70.

[39] Watson CP, Tyler KL, Bickers DR, et al. A randomized vehicle controlled trial of topical capsaicin in the treatment of postherpetic neuralgia. Clin Ther 1993;15:510–26.

[40] Watson CP, Evans R, Watt VR. Post herpetic neuralgia and topical capsaicin. Pain 1988; 33:333–40.

[41] Low PA, Opfer-Gehrking TL, Dyck PJ, et al. Double blind, placebo controlled study of the application of capsaicin cream in chronic distal painful polyneuropathy. Pain 1995;45: 163–8.

[42] Epstein JB, Marcoe JH. Topical application of capsaicin for treatment of oral neuropathic pain and trigeminal neuralgia. Oral Surg Oral Med Oral Pathol 1994;77: 135–40.

[43] Ellison N, Loprinzi CL, Kugler J, et al. Phase III placebo controlled trial of capsaicin cream in the management of surgical neuropathic pain in cancer patients. J Clin Oncol 1997;15: 2974–80.

[44] Morgenlander JC, Hurwitz BJ, Massey EW. Capsaicin for the treatment of pain in Guillain-Barré syndrome. Ann Neurol 1990;12:199.

[45] Turnbull A. Tincture of capsicum as a remedy for chilblains and toothache. Dublin (Ireland): Dublin Medical Press; 1850. p. 95–6.

[46] Altman RD, Aven A, Holmburg CE, et al. Capsaicin cream 0.025% as monotherapy for osteoarthritis: a double blind study. Sem Arth Rheum 1994;23S:25–33.

[47] Deal CL. The use of topical capsaicin in managing arthritis pain: a clinician's perspective. Sem Arth Rheum 1994;23S:48–52.

[48] Deal CL, Schnitzer TJ, Lipstein E, et al. Treatment of arthritis with topical capsaicin: a double blind trial. Clin Ther 1991;13:383–95.

[49] McCarthy GM, McCarty DJ. Effect of topical capsaicin in the therapy of painful osteoarthritis of the hands. J Rheumatol 1992;19:604–7.

[50] McCleane GJ. The analgesic efficacy of topical capsaicin in enhanced by glyceryl trinitrate in painful osteoarthritis: a randomized, double-blind, placebo controlled study. Eur J Pain 2000;4:355–60.

[51] Schnitzer T, Morton C, Coker S. Topical capsaicin therapy for osteoarthritis pain: achieving a maintenance regimen. Sem Arth Rheum 1994;23S:34–40.

[52] Mathias BJ, Dillingham TR, Zeigler DN, et al. Topical capsaicin for chronic neck pain. Am J Phys Med Rehabil 1995;74:39–44.

[53] Fitzgerald M. Capsaicin and sensory neurones. Pain 1983;15:109–30.

[54] Rains C, Bryson HM. Topical capsaicin. A review of its pharmacological properties and therapeutic potential in post herpetic neuralgia, diabetic neuropathy and osteoarthritis. Drugs Aging 1995;7:317–28.

[55] Nolano M, Simone DA, Wendelschafer-Crabb G, et al. Topical capsaicin in humans: parallel loss of epidermal nerve fibers and pain sensation. Pain 1999;81:135–41.

[56] Walker RA, McCleane GJ. The addition of glyceryl trinitrate to capsaicin cream reduces the thermal allodynia associated with the use of capsaicin in humans. Neurosci Lett 2002;323:78–80.

[57] McCleane GJ, McLaughlin M. The addition of GTN to capsaicin cream reduces the discomfort associated with application of capsaicin alone. A volunteer study. Pain 1998;78: 149–51.

[58] Yosipovitch G, Mailback HI, Rowbotham MC. Effect of EMLA pre-treatment on capsaicin-induced burning and hyperalgesia. Acta Derm Venereol 1999;79:118–21.

[59] Sawynok J. Adenosine receptor activation and nociception. Eur J Pharmacol 1998;317: 1–11.

[60] Esser MJ, Sawynok MJ. Caffeine blockade of the thermal antihyperalgesic effect of acute amitriptyline in a rat model of neuropathic pain. Eur J Pharmacol 2000;399:131–9.

[61] Sudoh Y, Cahoon EE, Gerner P, et al. Tricyclic antidepressant as long acting local anesthetics. Pain 2003;103:49–55.

[62] Haderer A, Gerner P, Kao G, et al. Cutaneous analgesia after transdermal application of amitriptyline versus lidocaine in rats. Anesth Analg 2003;96:1707–10.

[63] Esser MJ, Sawynok J. Acute amitriptyline in a rat model of neuropathic pain: differential symptom and route effects. Pain 1999;80:643–53.

[64] Esser MJ, Chase T, Allen GV, et al. Chronic administration of amitriptyline and caffeine in a rat model of neuropathic pain: multiple interactions. Eur J Pharmacol 2001;430: 211–8.

[65] Sawynok J, Esser MJ, Reid AR. Peripheral antinociceptive actions of desipramine and fluoxetine in an inflammatory and neuropathic pain test in the rat. Pain 1999;82:149–58.

[66] Sawynok J, Reid AR, Esser MJ. Peripheral antinociceptive action of amitriptyline in the rat formalin test: involvement of adenosine. Pain 1999;80:45–55.

[67] Sawynok J, Reid A. Peripheral interactions between dextromethorphan, ketamine and am-itriptyline on formalin-evoked behaviours and paw edema in rats. Pain 2003;102:179–86.

[68] Heughan CE, Allen GV, Chase TD, et al. Peripheral amitriptyline suppresses formalin-induced Fos expression in the rat spinal cord. Anesth Analg 2002;94:427–31.

[69] Su X, Gebhart GF. Effects of tricyclic antidepressants on mechanosensitive pelvic nerve afferent fibers innervating the rat colon. Pain 1998;76:105–14.

[70] Oatway M, Reid A, Sawynok J. Peripheral antihyperalgesic and analgesic actions of ket-amine and amitriptyline in a model of mild thermal injury in the rat. Anesth Analg 2003; 97:168–73.

[71] McCleane GJ. Topical doxepin hydrochloride reduces neuropathic pain: a randomized, double-blind, placebo controlled study. Pain Clin 1999;12:47–50.

[72] McCleane GJ. Topical application of doxepin hydrochloride, capsaicin and a combination of both produces analgesia in chronic human neuropathic pain: a randomized, double-blind, placebo-controlled study. Br J Clin Pharmacol 2000;49:574–9.

[73] Lynch ME, Clarke AJ, Sawynok J. A pilot study examining topical amitriptyline, ketamine, and a combination of both in the treatment of neuropathic pain. Clin J Pain 2003;19:323–8.

[74] McCleane GJ. Topical application of doxepin hydrochloride can reduce the symptoms of complex regional pain syndrome: a case report. Injury 2002;33:88–9.

[75] Epstein JB, Truelove EL, Oien H, et al. Oral topical doxepin rinse: analgesic effect in pa-tients with oral mucosal pain due to cancer or cancer therapy. Oral Oncol 2001;37:632–7.

[76] Zhou S, Komak S, Du J, et al. Metabotropic glutamate 1α receptors on peripheral primary afferent fibers: their role in nociception. Brain Res 2001;913:18–26.

[77] Carlton SM, Hargett GL, Coggeshall RE. Localization and activation of glutamate recep-tors in unmyelinated axons of rat glabrous skin. Neurosci Lett 1995;197:25–8.

[78] Carlton SM, Coggeshall RE. Inflammation-induced changes in peripheral glutamate recep-tor populations. Brain Res 1999;820:63–70.

[79] Zhou S, Bonasera L, Carlton SM. Peripheral administration of NMDA, AMPA or KA results in pain behaviour in rats. Neuroreport 1996;7:895–900.

[80] Jackson DL, Graff CB, Richardson JD. Glutamate participates in the peripheral modula-tion of thermal hyperalgesia in rats. Eur J Pharmacol 1995;284:321–5.

[81] Lawland NB, Willis WD, Westlund KN. Excitatory amino acid receptor involvement in peripheral nociceptive transmission in rats. Eur J Pharmacol 1997;324:169–77.

[82] Walker K, Reeve A, Bowes M, et al. mGlu5 receptors and nociceptive function II. mGlu5 receptors functionally expressed on peripheral sensory neurones mediate inflammatory hyperalgesia. Neuropharmacology 2001;40:10–9.

[83] Tverskoy M, Oren M, Vaskovich M, et al. Ketamine enhances local anesthetic and analge-sic effects of bupivicaine by a peripheral mechanism: a study in postoperative patients. Neurosci Lett 1996;215:5–8.

[84] Warncke T, JØrum E, Stubhaug A. Local treatment with the N-methyl-D-aspartate recep-tor antagonist ketamine, inhibits development of secondary hyperalgesia in man by a peripheral action. Neurosci Lett 1997;227:1–4.

[85] Pedersen JL, Galle TS, Kehlet H. Peripheral analgesic effects of ketamine in acute inflam-matory pain. Anesthesiology 1998;89:58–66.

[86] Hirota K, Lambert DG. Ketamine: its mechanism(s) of action and unusual clinical uses. Br J Anaesth 1996;77:441–4.

[87] Meller ST. Ketamine: relief from chronic pain through actions at the NMDA receptor? Pain 1996;68:435–6.

[88] Sawynok J, Reid AR. Modulation of formalin-induced behaviours and edema by local and systemic administration of dextromethorphan, memantine and ketamine. Eur J Pharmacol 2002;450:115–21.

[89] Crowley KL, Flores JA, Hughes CN, et al. Clinical application of ketamine ointment in the treatment of sympathetically maintained pain. Int J Pharmaceutical Compounding 1998;2: 122–7.

[90] Wood RM. Ketamine for pain in hospice patients. Int J Pharmaceutical Compounding
      2000;4:253–4.

[91] Davis CL, Treede RD, Raja SN, et al. Topical application of clonidine relieves hyperalgesia
      in patients with sympathetically maintained pain. Pain 1991;47:309–17.

[92] Epstein JB, Grushka M, Le N. Topical clonidine for orofacial pain: a pilot study. J Orofac
      Pain 1997;11:346–52.

[93] Torebjörk E, Wahren L, Wallin G, et al. Noradrenaline-evoked pain in neuralgia. Pain
      1995;63:11–20.

[94] Ali Z, Raja SN, Wesselmann U, et al. Intradermal injection of norepinephrine evokes pain
      in patients with sympathetically maintained pain. Pain 2000;88:161–8.

[95] Chabal C, Jacobson L, Mariano A, et al. The use of oral mexiletine for the treatment of pain
      after peripheral nerve injury. Anesthesiology 1992;76:513–7.

[96] Choi B, Rowbotham MC. Effect of adrenergic receptor activation on post-herpetic neural-
      gia pain and sensory disturbances. Pain 1997;69:55–63.

[97] Gentili M, Houssel P, Osman H, et al. Intra-articular morphine and clonidine produce com-
      parable analgesia but the combination is not more effective. Br J Anaesth 1997;79:660–1.

[98] Gentili M, Juhel A, Bonnet F. Peripheral analgesic effect of intra-articular clonidine. Pain
      1996;64:593–6.

[99] Reuben SS, Connelly NR. Postoperative analgesia for outpatient arthroscopic knee surgery
      with intraarticular clonidine. Anesth Analg 1999;88:729–33.

[100] Joshi M, Reuben SS, Kilaru PR, et al. Postoperative analgesia for outpatient arthroscopic
      knee surgery with intraarticular clonidine and/or morphine. Anesth Analg 2000;90:
      1102–6.

[101] Buerkle H, Huge V, Wolfgart M, et al. Intra-articular clonidine analgesia after knee
      arthroscopy. Eur J Anaesthesiol 2000;17:295–9.

[102] Calignano A, La Ranna G, Giuffrida A, et al. Control of pain initiation by endogenous
      cannabinoids. Nature 1998;394:277–81.

[103] Richardson JD, Kilo S, Hargreaves KM. Cannabinoids reduce hyperalgesia and inflamma-
      tion via interaction with peripheral CB1 receptors. Pain 1998;75:111–9.

[104] Fox A, Kesingland A, Gentry C, et al. The role of central and peripheral cannabinoid$_1$ re-
      ceptors in the antihyperalgesic activity of cannabinoids in a model of neuropathic pain.
      Pain 2001;92:91–100.

[105] Rice AS, Farquhar-Smith WP, Nagy I. Endocannabinoids and pain: spinal and peripheral
      analgesia in inflammation and neuropathy. Prostaglandins Leukot Essent Fatty Acids
      2002;66:243–56.

[106] Zhou L, Zhang Q, Stein C, et al. Contribution of opioid receptors on primary afferent ver-
      sus sympathetic neurons to peripheral opioid analgesia. J Pharmacol Exp Ther 1998;286:
      1000–6.

[107] Stein C, Schafer H, Hassan AH. Peripheral opioid receptors. Ann Med 1995;27:219–21.

[108] Coggeshall RE, Zhou S, Carlton SM. Opioid receptors on peripheral sensory axons. Brain
      Res 1997;764:126–32.

[109] Hassan AH, Ableitner A, Stein C, et al. Inflammation of the rat paw enhances axonal trans-
      port of opioid receptors in the sciatic nerve and increases their density in the inflamed tissue.
      Neuroscience 1993;55:185–95.

[110] Cerchietti LC, Navigante AH, Bonomi MR, et al. Effect of topical morphine for mucositis-
      associated pain following concomitant chemoradiotherapy for head and neck carcinoma.
      Cancer 2002;95:2230–6.

[111] Cerchietti LC, Navigante AH, Körte MW, et al. Potential utility of the peripheral analgesic
      properties of morphine in stomatitis-related pain: a pilot study. Pain 2003;105:265–73.

[112] Krajnik M, Zylicz Z, Finlay I, et al. Potential uses of topical opioids in palliative care—
      report of 6 cases. Pain 1999;80:121–5.

[113] Twillman RK, Long TD, Cathers TA, et al. Treatment of painful skin ulcers with topical
      opioids. J Pain Symptom Manage 1999;17:288–92.

[114] Likar R, Sittl R, Gragger K, et al. Peripheral morphine analgesia in dental surgery. Pain 1998;76:145–50.

[115] Likar R, Koppert W, Blatnig H, et al. Efficacy of peripheral morphine analgesia in inflamed, non-inflamed perineural tissue of dental surgery patients. J Pain Symptom Manage 2001;21:330–7.

[116] Moore RJ, Seymour RA, Gilro J, et al. The efficacy of locally applied morphine in postoperative pain after bilateral third molar surgery. Br J Clin Pharmacol 1994;37:227–30.

[117] Duckett JW, Cangiano T, Cubina M, et al. Intravesical morphine analgesia after bladder surgery. J Urol 1997;157:1407–9.

[118] McCoubrie R, Jeffrey D. Intravesical diamorphine for bladder spasm. J Pain Symptom Manage 2003;25:1–2.

[119] Picard PR, Tramer MR, McQuay HJ, et al. Analgesic efficacy of peripheral opioids (all except intra-articular): a qualitative systematic review of randomised controlled trials. Pain 1997;72:309–18.

[120] Gupta A, Bodin L, Holmstrom B, et al. A systematic review of the peripheral analgesic effects of intraarticular morphine. Anesth Analg 2001;93:761–70.

ELSEVIER
SAUNDERS

THE MEDICAL
CLINICS
OF NORTH AMERICA

Med Clin N Am 91 (2007) 141–167

Complementary and Alternative Medicine for Noncancer Pain

Gira Patel, LicAc[a], David Euler, LicAc[b],
Joseph F. Audette, MA, MD[c],*

[a]Osher Integrative Care Center, Harvard Medical School, Osher Institute,
Division for Research and Education in Complementary and Integrative Medical Therapies,
Kiiko Matsumoto International, 1647 Washington Street, Newton, MA 02465, USA
[b]Harvard Medical School, Kiiko Matsumoto International,
1647 Washington Street, Newton, MA 02465, USA
[c]Department of Physical Medicine and Rehabilitation, Harvard Medical School,
125 Nashua Street, Boston, MA 02114, USA

In most modern, allopathic Western pain clinics, patients are being treated with a multitude of medications and procedures that often create a vicious cycle of pain and adverse side effects. Patients are mostly treated symptomatically with medications that can be addictive in nature and procedures that often are not proven to be effective, all of which can cause a barrage of unwanted side effects. It is not uncommon that patients find themselves with a growing list of medications to take on a daily basis without experiencing true relief of pain or a return to a normal lifestyle. The problem has two sides, as many patients who come to pain clinics are seeking (and often demanding) quick fixes without the motivation or interest to devote any time or effort into a change in lifestyle and behavior that could often have a more profound effect on pain than what the clinician can provide. These patients expect (often unrealistically) the physician to diagnose and prescribe a medication or perform a procedure that eliminates the pain quickly even in a chronic condition and thereby absolves the patient of any responsibility to change. Unfortunately, physicians are often all too ready to make such heroic attempts, even when they know the attempt is unlikely to succeed, at the expense of patient wellness. In this pain management quagmire, complementary and alternative medicine (CAM) can provide a perfect

* Corresponding author. Spaulding Rehabilitation Hospital, 125 Nashua Street, Boston, MA 02114, USA
  E-mail address: jaudette@partners.org (J.F. Audette).

counterbalance to conventional approaches to help reintroduce a model of care that is more process oriented and helps move the patient from passive therapies to a more active role in their self care.

The National Center for Complementary and Alternative Medicine (NCCAM) is a US government agency dedicated to exploring complementary and alternative healing practices in the context of rigorous science, training CAM researchers, and disseminating authoritative information to the public and professionals. NCCAM defines complementary and alternative medicine as "a group of diverse medical and health care systems, practices, and products that are not presently considered to be part of conventional medicine." It also defines integrative medicine as "[combining] mainstream medical therapies and CAM therapies for which there is some high-quality scientific evidence of safety and effectiveness" [1].

The various modalities of CAM are well positioned to create a more healthy bridge between the patients' needs and the Western allopathic approaches. On one hand CAM approaches try to enhance and simplify the allopathic treatments as well as making them less toxic to the patient; on the other hand they try to engage the patients in their own healing process. Some of the more accepted and known CAM approaches include Traditional Chinese Medicine (TCM), which includes acupuncture and herbal formulas, Ayurveda (traditional Indian medicine), homeopathy, mind-body interventions (meditation, prayer, hypnosis, and so forth), vitamin and Western herbal approaches, chiropractic, massage therapy, osteopathic manipulations, yoga, and Tai-Chi to name a few.

Currently patients use CAM therapies upon referral from a friend or colleague and much less often as a result of a referral by their physician or other Western allopathic health care provider. As a result of this referral system, the modality that patients choose is often not based on a true evaluation of their condition and body-mind needs, but rather on patient preferences.

This article will provide an insight into some of the main CAM modalities and their potential clinical use within pain management.

Acupuncture

Chinese theory

Acupuncture is one the most widely used of the CAM modalities for pain management. There are a growing number of hospitals that offer acupuncture through their pain clinics as well as a growing number of physician and nonphysician acupuncturists. In 2002 the National Health Institute showed that an estimated 8.2 million adults had used acupuncture as opposed to an estimated 2.1 million that had used it in 2001. Not only is the usage of this modality growing but there is a growing body of research to support its efficacy as well [1].

To understand how acupuncture can be used for the management of pain, one has to understand its origins and purpose. Different from Western allopathic medicine where the symptomatic presentation of pain is often treated via a medication or a procedure, Traditional Chinese Medicine (acupuncture and Chinese herbal formulas) treats the individual by focusing on the root cause of why the patient cannot heal. TCM is tailored to the individual and not necessarily the "disease."

Acupuncture is a medical procedure in which fine, filliform needles are inserted into specific areas in the body (acupuncture points) to achieve clinical results either by modulating the course of a disease or by symptomatically reducing objective and subjective findings. Acupuncture is commonly practiced in conjunction with a technique called moxibustion. Moxibustion is a thermal therapy in which a dried herb, *Artemisia vulgaris,* is burned at or above the skin to deliver a heat stimulus to an area or acupuncture point.

Acupuncture is a medical practice that originated in China at least 3000 years ago. There are archeological findings of metallic acupuncture needles that date back to the late Shang dynasty (1000 BC). With the development of the Chinese culture and civilization, from the time of the Spring-Autumn period (770–475 BC) onward, there appeared different schools of philosophical thought. It was during this period that the theories of Yin-Yang and Five Phases (fundamental philosophical theories that attempt to explain the basis of every occurrence in nature) were applied to medicine. The most important and influential work of this period is the Huang di Neijing (Yellow Emperor's Internal Classic), predominantly the work of a number of scholars and physicians living between the fifth and first centuries BC, explaining pathogeneses as well as the diagnostic and treatment modalities. From the third century AD onward, acupuncture became a more specialized discipline in China with many outstanding specialists and numerous valuable books written to enhance the field. Acupuncture as a medical discipline has spread to many countries throughout Asia, Europe, and America, and as a result many different forms of acupuncture have evolved. Although all disciplines of acupuncture are based on Chinese Classic texts, one may find a great number of different styles, including various Japanese styles, Korean Hand Acupuncture, and auricular acupuncture along with Traditional Chinese Acupuncture.

To understand the practice of acupuncture in all these traditions it is important to have a rudimentary understanding of the basis of TCM theory. One of the most important concepts in TCM is the concept of "qi." Qi (Chee) refers to an energy force in the body. There is no direct translation of this term into English. It is a force that allows for movement, growth, warmth, and development in the body. In good health, qi flows freely through the meridian system. An obstruction in the flow of qi can lead to a manifestation of disease and pain. According to TCM, acupuncture points are used to bring the body back into a state of equilibrium by balancing the flow of qi in the meridian system and through the organs. There are 14 major meridians in the body; these meridians can be understood as virtual lines along the body's surface on which acupuncture points are found.

Yin and Yang

The concept of Yin and Yang is a unique binary understanding of opposites that is used for differential diagnosis and treatment strategy planning. All existing phenomena can be described, explained, and further divided into the Yin-Yang concept. The basic properties of heat, brightness, activity, moving outward, moving upward, and hyper-function belong to the concept of Yang. The basic properties of coldness, darkness, stillness, moving inward, moving downward, and hypo-function belong to the concept of Yin. Yin and Yang oppose each other and at the same time have an interdependent relationship. Physically, the upper parts of the body, the exterior and dorsal aspects of the body are all considered as Yang. The lower parts of the body, the interior and ventral aspects of the body are all Yin. Physiologically, Yin can be viewed as cholinergic, parasympathetic, as well as the solid aspect of the body, while Yang can be viewed as adrenergic, sympathetic, as well as the functional aspect of the organism.

The organ system

In TCM, the organ system is organized somewhat differently than in Western bio-medical systems. Each organ is considered a concept or a system that is in charge of specific physiological functions and corresponds to a variety of aspects of the body. The Zang organs are "solid" and are Yin in nature, but the Fu organs are hollow and considered Yang in nature. Organ concepts according to TCM are written with a capital letter (such as Spleen, Triple Warmer, Heart, and so forth); organs and functions according to Western understanding and terminology are written in lower case. Tables 1 and 2 provide an overview of the correlations between the Zang-Fu organs, their main functions, area of control, and diagnostic meaning. The extraordinary organs do not actually fall under the Zang-Fu organ system and have functions outside the scope of this monograph. They are Brain, Marrow, Bones, Blood Vessels, and Uterus.

Pathogenic causes of disease

The main categories for the differential diagnosis of a clinical presentation are called "Pathogenic Factors." These borrow their metaphors from nature and describe the manner in which a disease invades the body as well as the way it manifests in the individual patient. The actual symptomatic presentation of a disease is the interaction between the individual constitution and the pathogenic factor (see Table 3). Understanding these categories helps devise an herbal or acupuncture treatment.

Table 1
The five Zang Organs

Zang (Yin) Organ	Related Fu (Yang) Organ	Main Function	Opens Into:	Manifests On:	Related Function
Liver	Gallbladder	Maintaining potency and free flow of Qi	Eyes	Nails	Controls tendons, stores the blood
Heart	Small Intestine	Dominates the vessels	Tongue	Face	Houses the Mind, controls blood vessels
Spleen	Stomach	Governs digestion and assimilation	Mouth	Lips	Controls muscles, prevents prolapse of organs or extravasation of fluids
Lungs	Large Intestine	Circulates Qi and controls respiration	Nose	Body hair and skin	Dominates water dispersing, descending, hair, skin, and pores
Kidney	Urinary Bladder	Stores essence, regulates development and reproduction	Ear	Head hair	Dominates water metabolism, bone, teeth and the anterior and posterior orifices; manufactures marrow

Wind is a primary pathogenic factor as well as a carrier of other pathogens into the body as it invades. Because of its Yang nature, it tends to attack the posterior aspect and outer surfaces of the body first. However, it may quickly penetrate more deeply and progress into serious diseases if it is not expelled when it first attacks. Diseases caused by Wind are usually associated with external conditions, ie, colds and flu, intermittent symptoms, and migrating symptoms, ie, rheumatic arthritis, or abdominal pain that moves from one location to another. Wind diseases are usually rapid in onset; however, Wind can linger in the body for long periods of time and progress if undiagnosed or treated improperly. Wind can carry Heat, Cold, and Dampness; Wind can be external as well as internal in origin.

Wind-Heat is a syndrome associated with an "external pathogen." This is another way of saying the patient has a virus, like a common cold or a bacterial infection. The symptoms would be fever, chills, sore throat, and so forth. Wind-Cold is also an exterior pathogen, but is more likely to be a viral attack. Generally speaking, it is not common to see any kind of bacterial infections from an external influence represent as anything of a cold nature. This patient will have predominant chills, milder fever, and usually suffer from strong headache and body aches. Wind-Cold is differentiated from

Table 2
The six Fu Organs

Fu (Yang) Organ	Related Zang Organ	Main function
Gallbladder	Liver	Storing bile
Small Intestine	Heart	Separates the pure from the turbid
Stomach	Spleen	Receives and decomposes food
Large Intestine	Lung	Receives waste material sent down from the Small Intestine, absorbs its fluid content, and forms the remainder into feces for excretion
Urinary Bladder	Kidney	Temporary storage of urine
San-Jiao*	Pericardium	Govern various forms of Qi and assists in the passage of Yuan Qi and body fluid

* This Organ system is a description of functions without any form. The "Triple Warmer" is also a division of the body into three sections: Upper section (chest), Middle section (epigastric region to umbilicus), and Lower section (pelvic organs).

Wind-Heat by the patients' longing for hot drinks and cover. Wind-Damp is usually represented by arthritic disorders because the Wind combines with Dampness and it settles in the joints. Arthritic disorders are then further differentiated into Wind-Damp, Wind-Damp-Cold, and Wind-Damp-Heat. Internal Wind may be internally generated from a deficiency of Yin and/or Blood, or excessive Fire in the body. A few examples of internally generated Wind are epilepsy, convulsions, abnormal eye movements as with nystagmus, hypertension, tremor, or fitful movements.

Cold is a Yin pathogenic factor. If overly predominant, coldness can injure Yang, as Yang is hot and moving in nature; therefore, too much coldness can slow down the body's metabolic rate and create stagnation and pain, as well as fatigue and actual feeling of coldness. Coldness can be generated from an external influence, such as exposure to excessively cold conditions, or from an internal influence, such as eating or drinking too many cold (and raw) substances. Conversely, an excessive amount of Cold can accumulate from a deficient amount of qi and Yang in the body.

Heat is a Yang pathogenic factor. If overly predominant, Heat can injure Yin and cause dryness, inflammation, and pain. As Yin is lubricating and cooling in nature, deficiency of Yin ("Empty Heat") can stem from chronic disease, medications (or radiation), improper nutrition, too much processed sugar, and lack of hydration.

Dampness is heavy and turbid in nature. It therefore creates a blockage of energy wherever it settles in the body. This kind of blockage creates a heavy sensation. It may be a sensation of denseness, dullness, achiness, or even numbness. Dampness may also create such symptoms as turbid fluids in, or discharged from, the body, ie, excessive phlegm, discharge from the eyes, edema, or mucous in the stools, infection, and so forth. These

Table 3
Summary of potential pathological factors

Six external factors	The seven emotions	Miscellaneous factors
Wind	Joy	Improper diet
Cold	Anger	Over strain
Summer-Heat	Worry	Stress
Dampness	Pensiveness	Lack of exercise
Dryness	Sadness	Excessive sexual activity
Fire	Fear	Phlegm retention
	Shock	Blood stasis

discharges will often have a heavy, turbid type of odor. The patient with this pathogen will feel sluggish, and if the digestion is affected, abdominal distention and bloating will occur.

Dryness consumes body fluids. This condition may be contracted by external forces (if accompanied by Wind) but is more commonly seen as a result of a deficiency of fluids in the body due to chronic diseases, inflammation, and dehydration. Symptoms that may be associated can cause vascular disease, burning pain, wounds, and sores. Heat may come from dryness and includes chapped lips, dry skin, dry hair, excessive thirst, dry eyes, dry cough, and so forth.

Emotions may have an effect on the Organ it corresponds to or, conversely, may be an expression of the disease in an Organ system. The concept of emotional factors causing illness is common to both Western and Eastern traditions, but in Chinese Medicine, emotionally based diseases are not considered less real when compared with the "true" organ-based pathology we tend to do in the West. Clinically it is interesting to see that most patients' dominant emotion corresponds to the organ that is unbalanced. Generally speaking, the more severe the organ pathology or imbalance, the more expressive or strong the correspondent emotion may be.

According to TCM, the factor that is most likely to cause pain syndromes is called **Stagnation**. Several forms of Stagnation exist, such as stagnation of Qi, Blood, or Dampness and Phlegm. The differential diagnosis is based on the nature and quality of the pain. (A good article on the differential diagnosis of pain according to TCM is written by Giovanni Maciocia and can be found at http://www.giovanni-maciocia.com/articles/pain.html.) Qi Stagnation is the mildest form of pain and Blood stagnation the most severe. Acupuncture and Chinese herbal medicine are geared toward alleviating the Stagnation and reducing the pain.

Modern theory

Over the past 30 years, a great deal of scientific evidence has accumulated to verify that both Acupuncture Stimulation (AP) and Electro-Acupuncture Stimulation (EA) have reproducible physiological effects. There are two main lines of evidence that will be presented in the following paragraphs.

All go to the heart of the neurological mechanisms that are currently understood to modulate and influence pain.

A large body of evidence has developed to show that both AP and EA lead to the release of endorphins and enkephalins into the cerebrospinal fluid (CSF). Furthermore, the release of these neuropeptides has been demonstrated to play a role in the analgesic effect of acupuncture as evidenced by the fact that opioid receptor antagonism can abolish the analgesia obtained with acupuncture in both human and animal models of acute pain. There is evidence to support that the Hypothalamic-Pituitary Axis are also influenced by EA and AP and may further influence the analgesic response to pain both through immune modulation and modulation of the sympathetic responses, respectively. In addition, the release of 5-hydroxytryptamine (5HTP) has been demonstrated with AP and EA in the raphe nucleus and contributes to the analgesia presumably through descending inhibitory control mechanisms. Both the parameters of stimulation (ie, the intensity and frequency of EA) and the site of stimulation have significant effects on the type of chemical releases. In general, low-frequency (2 to 4 Hz), high-intensity stimulation such as with manual acupuncture or EA produces a slow in onset, cumulative affect on pain and is at least in part mediated through the endogenous opioid system; whereas, low-intensity, high-frequency stimulation (>70 Hz) produces a more rapid onset of pain relief that is partly mediated through the serotonin system [2].

The second line of evidence depends on recent technological advances in mapping brain activity using functional magnetic resonance scanning (fMRI) that have begun to be applied to acupuncture to demonstrate the neuromodulatory effect of acupuncture stimulation. Comparison has been made between tactile sensation (tapping the skin with a wire at 2 Hz) and AP using a manual stimulation technique. The acupuncture stimulation used in this study involves twisting the needle at 2 Hz in Large Intestine 4 (a point in the first dorsal interosseous muscle of the hand). Stimulation of an acupuncture point in this manner produces a deqi; a sensation that is a full, aching feeling at the point of the needle and is believed to be important in obtaining the clinical effect with AP. The results of unilateral AP showed bilateral neural modulation of cortical and subcortical structures, causing a signal decrease in the limbic region and other subcortical areas. Tactile stimulation did not produce these changes in fMRI [3].

Clinical data

The following is a summary of favorable, high-quality research papers on acupuncture and the treatment of common pain conditions.

Fibromyalgia

Signs and symptoms of fibromyalgia (FMS) can vary, depending on the weather, stress, physical activity, or even the time of day. The manifestation of this disorder varies from patient to patient, making it difficult to treat. Often patients suffering from fibromyalgia are highly sensitive and do not do well with current allopathic Western treatment strategies. A growing number of these patients turn to CAM therapies, of which acupuncture is one of the more popular choices. Berman and colleagues [4] reviewed seven studies, including three randomized controlled trials (RCTs) and four cohort studies; only one was of high methodological quality. The high-quality study suggests that acupuncture is effective for relieving pain, increasing pain thresholds, improving global ratings, and reducing morning stiffness of FMS; unfortunately the duration of benefit following the acupuncture treatment series is not known. The three lower-quality studies showed results consistent with these findings.

Shoulder pain

A recent high-quality study showed that acupuncture is an effective treatment for soft tissue lesions of the shoulder, including rotator cuff tendonitis, capsulitis, bicipital tendonitis, or bursitis [5]. This RCT included 130 patients divided into an acupuncture group and a placebo acupuncture group. Both groups were assessed before, during, and after procedure at 3 months and 6 months. After 6 months the true acupuncture group demonstrated statistically significant improvement over the placebo acupuncture group in the pain intensity score as well as range of motion, functionality, quality of life, and use of anti-inflammatory medication.

Epicondylitis

Trinh and colleagues [6] did a systematic review of 53 studies demonstrating that acupuncture was effective for short-term relief of lateral epicondyle pain. They identified six high-quality randomized or quasi-randomized trials that used needle acupuncture. The studies evaluated patients with any pain originating from the common extensor tendon at the lateral epicondyle. The acupuncture group in all six studies showed a significant relief in pain compared with the control group.

Headache

In 2001 a Cochrane Database review concluded that acupuncture had value in the treatment of idiopathic headache but that further high-quality studies were needed [7]. In recent years, better-designed studies have provided positive results for the treatment of chronic headaches and migraines. In a RCT of 270 patients, Melchart and colleagues [8] concluded that acupuncture had an effect comparable to other types of Western allopathic headache treatments. In another RCT of 302 patients suffering from migraines [9], the patients were divided into three groups: true or verum acupuncture, sham acupuncture, and waiting list control. Sham acupuncture was defined as superficial needling at distant nonacupuncture points. The result of this study was similar to that of Melchart and colleagues in that the number of days with headache was significantly reduced in the acupuncture and sham acupuncture group compared with that of the waiting list. However, the sham treatment was as effective as the true acupuncture treatment.

Another long-term randomized controlled trial studied patients with chronic headaches (the majority had migraines) at baseline, 3 months, and 12 months [10]. At the end of a year the study showed that the patients who received acupuncture had significantly lower headache scores than the control group. In addition, the acupuncture group missed fewer days from work, used less medication, and had fewer visits to the general practitioner than did patients in the control group. A smaller study was performed to study the change in cerebrovascular blood flow in patients suffering from migraine headaches [11]. This study showed that 60% of migraineurs in the trial who benefited from the acupuncture had less abnormality in cerebrovascular response to visual stimulation.

Neck pain

Neck pain (as well as low back pain) is one of the most common symptoms for which patients seek CAM therapies. Irnich and colleagues [12] published a randomized, double-blinded, sham-controlled, crossover trial investigating the effect of acupuncture on patients with chronic neck pain. The patients included in this study presented with at least a 2-month history of neck pain with limited range of motion (ROM) and active myofascial trigger points. The patients were divided into three groups: nonlocal acupuncture (acupuncture given in points distal to the presenting complaint of neck pain), dry needling (local dry needling of the active trigger points in the neck), and sham laser acupuncture. Each patient was given one 30-minute session and then assessed. The study concluded that a single session of nonlocal acupuncture was superior to dry needling and sham laser to immediately improve motion-related cervical pain and ROM. The results of this study suggest that stimulation of distal points on the body can be more effective than local needling for short-term pain relief, supporting the concept that nonsegmental antinociceptive systems may play a major role in acupuncture analgesia. In another very large study done in Germany with 14,161 patients, subjects with chronic neck pain were randomized to acupuncture or a control group with no acupuncture [13]. In addition, all patients were allowed to receive usual medical care. At 3 months, patients in the acupuncture group had significant improvement in neck pain and disability over the control group. This study also demonstrates that acupuncture can be a valuable adjunct to usual medical care.

Pain during pregnancy

Elden and colleagues [14] conducted a randomized, single-blinded, controlled trial with 386 pregnant women suffering from pelvic girdle pain. The women were randomized into three groups: standard treatment, standard treatment with acupuncture, and standard treatment with stabilization exercises. The patients receiving acupuncture showed significantly lower pain scores when compared with patients receiving standard care alone or standard care with stabilization exercises. This study also demonstrated that using acupuncture in conjunction with standard Western allopathic care is more beneficial to a patient in a clinical setting. Another RCT showed acupuncture to be effective in decreasing visual analogue scale (VAS) pain scores in pregnant women suffering from low back pain and pelvic pain [15]. The study also reported decreases in pain during physical activity in the subjects who received acupuncture. These studies should help the physician practicing Western allopathic medicine to feel comfortable prescribing acupuncture for pregnant patients who suffer from pain.

Low back pain

A study published by the Cochrane Review that included 35 randomized controlled trials concluded that acupuncture is an effective treatment for chronic low back pain (LBP) [16]. A recent meta-analysis had similar conclusions, finding that acupuncture was effective in the relief of LBP [17]. This review not only supported the analgesic effect of acupuncture for LBP, but also suggests that acupuncture can improve functionality and lead to decreased use of analgesic medications in this population. These data are very encouraging and should lead to at least the consideration of using acupuncture rather than opioids to manage chronic LBP. Another study published in the *Archives of Internal Medicine* showed that patients who received acupuncture over an 8-week period had a greater reduction in low back pain than those on a waiting list control [18]. Molsberger and colleagues [19] demonstrated that acupuncture coupled with conventional orthopedic treatment (COT) was much more effective than COT alone or sham acupuncture with COT in relieving chronic low back pain.

Knee pain

In recent years a number of well-designed studies have been published, demonstrating the positive effect of acupuncture on knee osteoarthritis. A large RCT published by Berman and colleagues [20] showed that acupuncture provided significantly more pain relief and improvement of function in patients suffering from osteoarthritis of the knee. Another study by Linde and colleagues [21] showed that patients with various types of osteoarthritis demonstrated a decrease in pain for up to 6 months after acupuncture treatments. Acupuncture has also been shown to be a complementary therapy to pharmacological treatment [22]. Vas and colleagues [22] showed that patients who received acupuncture and diclofenac versus diclofenac and placebo acupuncture had a greater decrease in pain and stiffness. In addition, the group receiving true acupuncture had a significant increase in physical function.

Herbal medicine

Herbal medicine is the use of various parts of plants for medicinal purposes. Since the beginning of history all indigenous cultures in the world have used natural substances (especially plants and animal parts) to promote healing and alleviate pain. In the modern Western clinic, the most common approaches in herbal medicine include Western herbal approaches, traditional Chinese herbal formulas, and Ayurvedic medicine (traditional Indian medicine). This section will emphasize the Western and Traditional Chinese approaches.

The main difference in the various approaches to herbal medicine lies in the differential diagnosis and the clinical strategies for prescribing specific herbs. While in the Western approach the strategy for prescribing herbs is more symptom-oriented and leans toward single herbs for specific ailments, the Ayurvedic and Traditional Chinese approaches rely on prescribing herbal combinations (formulas) for syndromes as they appear in different types of patients. For example, a "hot patient" who presents with a red face, feeling warm, and might run a higher blood pressure as opposed to a "cold patient" who might present with a pale face and body, feeling cold, and have a lower blood pressure. This unique difference between approaches can be bridged in clinical practice by using the best of both worlds. For example, if a patient is suffering from chronic low back pain, one can prescribe an external rub of the essential oils from lavender (warming and analgesic) and rosemary (stimulating circulation) as well as a Traditional Chinese herbal formula, Te Xiao Yao Tong Pian (treating weak kidney qi with cold back and frequent urination as well as knee pain and impotence) taken internally as herbal pills.

As one can see the differential diagnosis for the Traditional Chinese herbal formula is more complex and requires an understanding of whether certain conditions are present in the patient in addition to the symptom of low back pain to make the prescription of this specific formula. Often one can find a multitude of Traditional Chinese herbal formulas for one specific symptom. This depends on the constitution of the patient, etiology of disease, and the coexistence of other symptomatic presentations such as heat or cold, dampness or dryness, or symptoms located mainly in the upper body or lower body. Also apparent, when one reads the indications of the Chinese herbal formulas, is that the language used for the differential diagnosis differs from that used in Western, allopathic medicine.

The Western approach to herbs treating pain syndromes is more symptom-oriented and restricted to single herb functions. Single herbs are often combined to treat one or several symptoms. The single herb approach is simpler to research and control, but the effects may not be as comprehensive and satisfactory or well-fitted to the individual patient as Chinese herbal formulas. Several herbs were found to have satisfactory analgesic effects, among them Rhizoma Curcumae (*Curcuma wenyujin, Curcuma phaeocaulis,* and *Curcuma kwangsiensis* are the three species of Curcuma rhizomes being used) [23–29], Ginger extract [30,31], Willow bark [32,33], Capsaicin [34–36], Devil's Claw, Boswellia [37–39] , Lavender [40–42] , and Feverfew [43,44]. Most commonly these herbal remedies are ingested in capsules that contain concentrated extracts of the herb. The essential oil of these herbs can be ingested, inhaled, or rubbed onto the painful area. For a milder effect, one can drink the tea or infusion of these herbs.

Manual therapies

Manipulative therapies

The use of manipulative therapies for spine-related pain is widespread and in recent surveys found to be one of the most highly used CAM therapies in the United States [45,46]. The origins of both chiropractic manipulation and osteopathic practices of spinal manipulative therapy (SMT) go back to the late nineteenth century, but with recent advances in the understanding of the physiology of pain, both schools of thought have moved beyond the concept of joint subluxation to theoretically ground their work. Panjabi [47] has advanced a biomechanical model of spinal pain that emphasizes the requirement of normal function in the active, passive, and neural integration systems of the spine as a prerequisite for stability. The loss of spinal stability occurs when one of the components of the active (musculotendinous), passive (ligamentous), and neural integration (proprioceptors, nociceptors) becomes dysfunctional. This is necessarily followed by compensations of the other systems. Such compensatory responses may trigger movement impairments, such as pain avoidance, or control impairments, such as pain provocation.

In addition to biomechanical models, neurophysiological mechanisms are often used to explain the diverse clinical effects of SMT, such as increased pain tolerance, reduced alpha-motor neuron activity, increased proprioceptive function, and autonomic modulation. Like acupuncture, SMT and other manual therapy interventions appear to have neurophysiological effects that can cause pain modulation. Both techniques are known to trigger similar populations of proprioceptive afferents (Groups I and II) that can gate nociception in the dorsal horn [48]. Either technique may activate the diffuse noxious inhibitory control system (DNIC) [49]. This is an antinociceptive or analgesic pathway activated over a short time period and triggered by nociceptive conditioning stimuli. This mechanism uses a nociceptive input to block pain in some other location.

Clinical data

There are more than 73 RCTs evaluating SMT, the vast majority of which are studies of chiropractic manipulation as opposed to osteopathic.

Most studies evaluated pain syndromes involving the low back, neck, and headaches. The designs varied from having placebo controls to comparisons with standard medical treatments. Meeker and Haldeman [50] have reviewed a total of 43 RCTs using SMT for acute, subacute, and chronic low back pain. Thirty of these RCTs favored SMT over the comparison treatment in at least one patient subgroup. The remaining 13 reported no significant differences, and none of the RCTs reported that SMT was less effective than the comparison treatment. Eight of the 11 placebo-controlled trials for low back pain favored the use of SMT. The results of SMT in the treatment of cervical spine pain have been mixed. Eleven RCTs have been conducted, four with positive results and seven that were equivocal. In the RCTs evaluating SMT for headache treatment, seven of the nine RCTs were positive. However, a review by Assendelft and colleagues [51] of 39 RCTs for acute and chronic LBP concluded that there was no clinical advantage seen in the literature to support chiropractic care over care by a primary care physician or a physical therapist and that analysis of study quality did not alter these results. For example, in an RCT of acute LBP, comparing chiropractic care to physical therapy or a self-care educational booklet, all three interventions led to improvement in pain and function at long-term follow-up, but there was no significant difference found between groups [52].

One of the issues that may affect the outcomes of these studies is correct patient selection. In a recent study, it was found that subjects responded significantly to spinal manipulation compared with a control exercise intervention if symptom duration was fewer than 16 days, there were no symptoms distal to knee, subjects had a score of less than 19 on a fear of movement avoidance measure [53], and they had at least one hypomobile lumbar segment and at least one hip with more than 35 degrees of internal rotation [54].

With regard to specific studies of osteopathic treatment of low back pain, there have been two recent studies, both with methodological flaws that have been published. Andersson and colleagues [55] performed a randomized, controlled trial that involved patients who had back pain for at least 3 weeks but less than 6 months. The patients were treated with either one or more standard medical therapies (72 patients) or with osteopathic manual therapy (83 patients). A variety of outcome measures were used, including the Roland–Morris and Oswestry questionnaires and a visual-analog pain scale, as well as objective measurements of range of motion and straight leg raise over a 12-week study period. Over the course of the study, patients in both groups improved. There was no statistically significant difference between the two groups in any of the primary outcome measures [55].

Williams and colleagues [56] looked at the effectiveness and health care costs of a practice-based osteopathy clinic for subacute spinal pain. The study included 201 patients with neck or back pain of 2 to 12 weeks' duration who were randomly assigned to usual care given by a general practitioner (GP) versus usual care with an additional three treatment sessions of osteopathic spinal manipulation. The primary outcome measure was the Extended Aberdeen Spine Pain Scale (EASPS). Secondary measures included SF-12, EuroQol, and Short-form McGill Pain Questionnaire. Health care costs were estimated from the records of referring GPs. Results of the study revealed that more patients improved who received the additional osteopathic treatment. At 2 months this improvement was significantly greater in EASPS, but at 6 months this difference was no longer significant for EASPS but remained significant for the SF-12 mental score. Mean health care costs attributed to spinal pain were significantly greater in the osteopathy group. Conclusions drawn were that a primary care osteopathy clinic improved short-term physical and longer psychological outcomes, with reasonable extra cost [56].

Adverse clinical events, such as cauda equina syndrome (CES) and vertebral artery dissection, have been difficult to evaluate, as the events are rare. This is especially true regarding vertebral artery dissection with subsequent cerebrovascular accident (CVA). None of the previously mentioned RCTs or any case series has reported a serious complication. In a Danish series, inclusive of 99% of chiropractors over a 10-year period, five cases of CVA and one death were identified [57]. One of the most comprehensive assessments of the complications of spinal manipulation was conducted by Koes and colleagues [58] in 1996 who identified relevant case reports, surveys and review articles using a comprehensive search of online databases. Based on case reports and surveys, estimation was made of the risk for the most frequently reported complications, which included vertebral basilar accidents (VBAs) and CES. They found that VBAs occurred mainly after a cervical manipulation with a rotatory component with an estimated occurrence of 1 per 20,000 patients to 1 per 1 million cervical manipulations. They reported the risk of CES to be one in a million. Based on malpractice claims, the prevalence of vertebral artery dissection and stroke following cervical manipulation is 1 case in 5.8 million. Estimates of the incidence of CES following lumbar manipulation range from 1 case per 100 million to 1 in 1 million [59].

Massage

A problem with studying the clinical effects of manual therapy is the significant nonspecific influence of touch on pain outcomes, separate from any specific details of the clinical technique used. It has been found in animal models that massage-like stroking of rats will increase withdrawal latencies in response to thermal and mechanical painful stimuli. This effect is in part related to the increased level of oxytocin in the periaquaductal gray (PAG) area of the midbrain that can be induced by touch. Oxytocin can influence descending antinociceptive systems via the PAG, and its effect can be attenuated by u and k opioid receptor antagonists [60].

Clinical data

There have been well-powered studies of massage in the pain literature for LBP and neck pain. Most trials compare massage to another CAM or conventional treatment rather than attempt to find a sham or placebo massage intervention.

A meta-analysis found three recent high-quality RCTs using massage for LBP [61]. One compared massage versus acupuncture or an educational booklet for LBP [62]; one compared massage to relaxation training [63]; and the final study compared massage versus exercise or a sham cold laser treatment [64]. The conclusion of the analysis was that massage appeared to provide a benefit for chronic LBP and may involve a cost savings compared with acupuncture or patient education.

There may be an added benefit when massage is combined with other treatments for LBP. In the study by Preyde [64] of 102 subjects with subacute to chronic LBP of fewer than 8 months' duration, subjects were randomized to either comprehensive massage, massage alone, an exercise regimen or a sham cold laser treatment. Each group was provided six treatments over a 1-month period with a 1-month posttreatment follow-up. At 1 month follow up, 63% of the comprehensive massage group were pain free, 27% in the massage alone, 14% in the exercise group, and 0% in the sham laser group. The comprehensive massage group involved the use of various soft tissue massage techniques, stretching exercises, and education about body mechanics.

There are two trials that compare a massage intervention to acupuncture, one for chronic neck pain and the other for chronic LBP. In the neck pain study, 177 subjects were randomized to either acupuncture, sham cold laser, or massage [65]. Each group received five treatments with assessment at 1 week posttreatment. There was significant improvement in pain in the acupuncture group when compared with massage and sham laser, with those diagnosed with myofascial neck pain showing the greatest improvement with acupuncture. In this study, the acupuncture included local treatment of myofascial trigger points in the neck using a dry needling method and did not rely exclusively on a Chinese formulaic treatment protocol. In contrast, a large RCT of 262 subjects with chronic LBP that compared a Traditional Chinese style of acupuncture to massage and a self-care education booklet found that only massage had significant positive effects on pain and function at 52-week follow-up [62].

There has been one poorly powered RCT of massage for fibromyalgia. In this study, 24 adult fibromyalgia patients were randomized to either massage or relaxation therapy [66]. Each subject received 30-minute treatments two times per week for 5 weeks. Outcomes included measurement of total sleep hours, pain, tender points, and salivary substance P levels. Only the subjects in the massage group had significant improvement in sleep hours, fewer tender points, and lower levels of substance P.

Movement therapies

Exercise or coordinated movement is an essential component of the treatment of a variety of musculoskeletal pain conditions. Exercise is one key management strategy used by physical therapists to address impairments (problems with body function or structure such as pain or weakness), activity limitations (difficulties an individual may have in executing activities such as walking, sitting, and standing), and participation restrictions (problems an individual may experience in life situations such as working, playing sports, or socializing) in patients with chronic pain. Multiple meta-analyses on the effects of exercise on various painful conditions report exercise to have a positive effect on pain, aerobic capacity, and physical function. The mechanisms behind these effects are not completely clear and are most likely attributable to multiple factors [67]. Exercise may also influence pain in a number of nonspecific ways, eg, through its influences on body mass, mood, sleep, motivation, deconditioning, skill acquisition, self-efficacy, or social contact.

Most studies have investigated whether decreased sensitivity to pain (hypoalgesia) occurs following aerobic exercise, with less research investigating whether hypoalgesia occurs after other modes of exercise (eg, resistance or isometric exercise). A number of investigators have reported the development of hypoalgesia during and following exercise under experimental and clinical conditions [68]. Hypoalgesia following exercise does appear to be mediated in part by the endogenous opioid system; however, an elevation in pain threshold can also occur following pre-injection with opioid antagonists, providing evidence for a nonopioid-based mechanism [69]. In addition to activation of large caliber sensory afferent fibers (A-β) with movement that can have a gating effect on pain, the small caliber sensory fibers in muscles have been shown to activate as well with exercise, which could lead to hypoalgesic effects potentially through diffuse noxious inhibitory control (DNIC) mechanisms similar to those outlined in the "manipulative and manual therapy" section [70].

The data to support CAM exercise methods, such as yoga and Tai Chi, for pain conditions is still sparse. Nevertheless, there are some recent studies that suggest that these alternative exercise modalities may play a more significant role in the future. In particular, yoga and Tai Chi incorporate movement and mindfulness into their discipline, which may make the hypoalgesic effect more potent, taking advantage of both mind-body and exercise-based influences on nociception.

Clinical data on yoga

There are now data to support the use of yoga in the treatment of chronic low back pain. Williams and colleagues [71] used Iyengar yoga in a 16-week, controlled trial of patients with more than 10 years of chronic low back pain. Univariate analyses of medical and functional outcomes recorded at 3-month follow-up found significant reductions in pain intensity (64%), functional disability (77%), and pain medication usage (88%) in the yoga group. In another recent study, Cherkin and colleagues [72] randomized 101 patients into three groups, giving one group yoga, a second physical therapy, and assigning the third control group a self-help book. Yoga outperformed the self-help book group on the Roland 24 scale at 12 and 26 weeks ($P <$ .001 in each case), and outperformed physical therapy on a "bothersomeness scale" at 12 weeks ($P < .001$).

Clinical data on Tai Chi

Recent studies suggest that Tai Chi (TCC) has been shown to be a safe method of exercise from a cardiovascular point of view and requires an energy expenditure that is equivalent to brisk walking [73]. This low-level aerobic effect may in itself have some hypoalgesic effect as stated above. We theorize that TCC practice provides cognitive training that is similar to that found with meditation-based stress-reduction techniques. Qigong breathing exercises have been recognized to have a similar physiologic effect as mind-body relaxation techniques and are often incorporated in TCC practice [74]. A small RCT of 33 patients with osteoarthritis reported that 12 weeks of Tai Chi practice significantly improved arthritis symptoms, self-efficacy, level of tension, and satisfaction with general health status [75]. Similar results were found in a larger RCT assessing the effect of TCC on 72 patients with osteoarthritic pain in a middle-aged and elderly population using shortened forms of the Sun-style of Tai Chi. The Tai Chi group perceived significantly less pain and stiffness in their joints and reported fewer perceived difficulties in physical functioning when compared with the control group after the 12-week exercise intervention [76].

Mind-body therapies

Meditation theory

Meditation is the most commonly researched and used form of mind-body therapy for pain. The focus of therapy is generally less upon the end of being pain-free and more upon becoming better able to cope with and manage pain, thereby improving one's level of functioning. In the United States today, the two most widely researched meditative practices by a wide margin are transcendental meditation or TM [77], often referred to as the "relaxation response" within the medical community, and mindfulness meditation. Most relaxation techniques [78,79], such as structured breathing exercises, guided imagery or visualization, hypnosis, biofeedback, autogenic training, repetitive prayer, certain forms of repetitive exercise or activity (eg, yoga, Tai Chi, and qi gong), all involve the reduction of muscle tension and a slowing down of normal physiological activity. These activities theoretically induce a hypometabolic state involving a parasympathetic response that will result in reduced heart rate, blood pressure, respiratory rate, and musculoskeletal tension [80]. As a result, they all may provide some measure of relief from chronic pain. What all these mind-body approaches have in common, according to Benson [78], is that they all involve (1) the repetition of a word, sound, mantra, phrase, or muscular activity, and (2) the passive disregard of everyday thoughts or distractions, with the subject returning to his or her repetition, whenever he or she becomes aware of having been distracted.

Meditation may be distinguished from other forms of deep relaxation, where the goal is often to exchange one set of mental contents for another, as in guided imagery or visualization, hypnosis, and autogenic training. Instead, meditation emphasizes alertness, [81,82] a state of expanded self-awareness with a heightened sense of integrated cohesion [83]. Meditation may also be contrasted with practices that involve repetitive exercise, such as yoga, Tai Chi, and qi gong, because it does not typically involve additional elements of structured breathing, postures, and scripts for movement that require bodily mastery that could detract from training attention and awareness [84].

Deep meditation can reduce cortisol secretion, oxygen consumption, and blood lactate levels, and increase the secretion of hormones such as serotonin and melatonin [83,85]. Until recently, it was thought that the relaxation response and mindfulness meditation exerted their therapeutic physiological influence by reducing sympathetic arousal and increasing the activity of the parasympathetic nervous system, thereby moderating the impact of chronic stress or the fight-or-flight response [86]. Recent studies of the neural basis of meditation, however, point to sharp increases in vasoconstrictor arginine vasopressin, resulting in decreased fatigue among meditators, as well as heightened arousal [81]. Research now indicates a mutual activation of the parasympathetic and sympathetic systems during meditation, as opposed to the original view of parasympathetic dominance, consistent with a balanced autonomic response that is, in turn, consistent with subjective descriptions of meditation as eliciting a sense of profound calmness as well as alertness and attunement [87].

Clinical data

The empirical literature suggests that mindfulness meditation may lead to reduced symptoms in a variety of problematic medical conditions and illnesses, including chronic pain, stress-related disorders, anxiety, depression, binge eating, fibromyalgia, and psoriasis, as well as ancillary symptoms associated with some forms of cancer and multiple sclerosis [88]. With meditation, chronic pain can be influenced positively through a variety of mechanisms and neural pathways, including changes in the quality of neurotransmission, generation of pain-blocking endorphins, evocation of pain-blocking positive emotions, selective redirection of attention away from the perception of pain, and adjustment of the spinal gateways to the brain.

Meditation, however, is difficult to standardize, quantify, and authenticate for research purposes. Issues of adherence and compliance among subjects, choice of beginner versus advanced practitioners, and reliance largely on self-report in many comparative or efficacy-effectiveness study designs all add to the methodological challenges involved in the scientific research of meditation [89]. True randomization of subjects exists in few studies, as meditators are typically a self-selected group. Selection bias and expectancy effects therefore represent powerful limitations in our ability to generalize conclusions to larger populations. Some researchers also point to a confounding longitudinal bimodal impact of meditation, with deep relaxation being elicited among beginners but with structurally more enduring hormonal and metabolic changes being detected among more experienced meditators [83].

Hypnosis

Hypnosis has been used for both acute and chronic pain conditions. In the chronic pain arena, the primary goal is not just to alter pain for a brief period during the hypnotic trance but to make hypnotic suggestions and teach skills that will alter pain intensity and its impact throughout the patient's daily life. Typical suggestions made during hypnosis include direct diminution of pain, relaxation, imagined analgesia, decreased pain unpleasantness, and replacement of pain with other nonpainful sensations or pain displacement (ie, moving the pain to other nonpainful areas of the body).

Theory

There are at least three mechanisms potentially involved in hypnotic analgesia: (1) sensory attenuation of nociception at the level of spinal cord, (2) reduction of the awareness of nociceptive input at higher centers, and (3) reduction in the experience of unpleasantness over and beyond reductions in pain sensation. Modern neuroimaging techniques provide additional experimental evidence to suggest that hypnosis influences pain-related changes in regional cerebral blood flow (rCBF) in the anterior cingulate cortex but not in the somatosensory cortex. This provides evidence that hypnosis-induced analgesia involves frontal-lobe limbic activity altering the emotional processing of pain [90,91]. In other imaging studies [92,93] it appears that hypnotic suggestions for decreased pain effectively reduced the unpleasantness of pain, particularly in highly hypnotizable individuals. Suggestions for increased pain affect influenced unpleasantness more than intensity, and this effect increased with repetition of the suggestions.

Clinical data

In a recent review of the use of hypnosis in chronic pain, the authors concluded that hypnotic analgesia produces significantly greater decreases in pain relative to no-treatment and to some nonhypnotic interventions, such as medication management, physical therapy, and education/advice. The most common chronic pain condition in the review was headache [94] with only one or two studies included in the review on low back pain, fibromyalgia, osteoarthritis, cancer-related pain, temporomandibular pain disorder, and mixed pain conditions. Interestingly when hypnosis was compared with other mind-body interventions, such as progressive muscle relaxation and autogenic training (both of which often include hypnotic-like suggestions), the positive effects of self-hypnosis training on chronic pain was similar. Patient expectancy about the positive benefits of hypnosis appeared to play a significant role in some of the studies in the review, and because a credible placebo treatment has not been developed, conclusions cannot yet be made about whether hypnotic analgesia treatment is specifically effective over and above its effects on expectancy. Finally, the review found that global hypnotic responsiveness and ability to experience vivid images are associated with positive treatment outcome in hypnosis, progressive relaxation, and autogenic training treatments [95].

In a controlled study comparing hypnosis to physical therapy, 40 subjects were randomly assigned to either eight 1-hour sessions of hypnotherapy (supplemented by a self-hypnosis home practice tape) over a 3-month period, or 12 to 24 hours of physical therapy (that included massage and muscle relaxation training) over a 3-month period. Outcome was assessed pretreatment, posttreatment, and at 3-month follow-up. The hypnosis intervention began with an arm levitation induction and included standard ego strengthening suggestions as well as suggestions for general relaxation, improved sleep, and "control of muscle pain." Larger improvements were found in the patients who received hypnosis than in those who received physical therapy on measures of muscle pain, fatigue, sleep disturbance, distress, and patient overall assessment of outcome, and these differences were maintained at 3-month follow-up. The average percent decrease in pain among patients who received hypnosis was 35% compared with a 2% decrease in the patients who received physical therapy [96].

In a study of chronic osteoarthritis pain, hypnosis was compared with a progressive muscle relaxation treatment condition and to a no-treatment control condition in 36 patients with osteoarthritis. The hypnosis treatment involved relaxation suggestions for the induction and then suggestions for pleasant memories involving the use of the joint when it was not painful. The relaxation condition was eight sessions of standard progressive muscle relaxation training. In this study, both interventions were more effective than no treatment, and there were no significant differences in outcome between the two active interventions overall. However, hypnosis did show a trend to be more effective than relaxation (56% average pre- to posttreatment improvement versus 31% improvement), and the difference in improvement between the two treatments was statistically significant at the mid-point (4 weeks after treatment began) of treatment. Patients in both treatment conditions also reported similar decreases in medication use over the course of treatment that was not observed in the no-treatment condition [97].

In a study of 66 patients with chronic migraine headaches, subjects were randomly assigned to one of five different experimental conditions: two hypnotic analgesia interventions, a hand temperature biofeedback condition, a relaxation training condition, and a 3-month standard care control condition. Participants in one of the hypnosis conditions were "instructed in self-hypnosis." Those in the second hypnosis condition were given the same instructions as those in the first condition but also given a hypnotic suggestion to visualize putting their hands in bowls of warm water. The hand temperature biofeedback condition included standard hypnotic-like autogenic suggestions. The relaxation response intervention involved "step-by-step" instruction in obtaining a relaxation response through mental repetition of a single word following Benson's model. All treatment subjects received three sessions of weekly treatment, and outcome was assessed pre- and post-treatment, as well as at 6-, 9-, and 12-month follow-up. The three outcome measures were peak headache pain intensity, number of headaches, and medication use, computed from data taken from 3-week periods of headache diaries completed just before each assessment point; standard care patients completed diaries for 3 months before being assigned to a treatment condition. Their results indicated that patients in both hypnosis groups showed greater decreases in all three outcome measures than these patients did during their 3-month period of standard care. The two hypnosis treatment interventions were no more effective, on average, than either relaxation response or the hand temperature biofeedback training conditions on any of the outcome measures [98].

In their review, Jensen and Patterson [95] conclude with suggestions for future research: (1) Can the effects of hypnotic analgesia treatment be accounted for by the effects of treatment on outcome expectancy? (2) Do the relative rates of responsiveness to hypnosis treatment differ as a function of pain type? (3) How should the problem of variability in hypnosis treatments between studies be dealt with when comparing study results? (4) What are the primary components of hypnotic analgesia interventions that contribute to their efficacy?

Summary

In summary, the past several years have shown an increase in the quality of trials examining the clinical efficacy of various CAM modalities for pain conditions. There is still need to raise the quality of the studies from a scientific and methodological point of view in many areas of CAM research by randomization, appropriate sample size, blinding, and developing more sophisticated sham procedures. However, much work still has to be done to find ways to preserve the clinical authenticity of CAM treatment methods when brought into the light of a research protocol. Recent attempts have been made to find a method of maintaining the standardization and reproducibility of research protocols while allowing the kind of flexible treatment that would normally be applied in a clinical setting. Other questions that should be answered with future studies include understanding how treatment length influences outcome, if maintenance treatments are needed for chronic conditions, and cost and risk comparisons with standard pharmacological treatment. Providing this kind of detail will assist both with reproducibility as well as help us gain a better understanding about whether certain treatment paradigms are superior to others for specific clinical conditions. Finally, physicians who have an interest in pursuing CAM research should educate themselves both about the methodological issues inherent with the particular area of interest as well as about ways to maintain the authenticity of the CAM treatment protocols so that the literature is not populated with more poorly designed studies. With the emerging interest in integrative medicine, there is a growing interest in collaboration and a greater number of physicians are interested in obtaining training in CAM modalities to help bridge this gap between CAM and conventional clinicians. For example, the American Academy of Medical Acupuncturists (AAMA) has been formed to help as both an educational and research forum for physician acupuncturists and the American Holistic Medical Association provides educational exposure in a broad range of Integrative and CAM modalities. The future of medicine will likely be Integrative and the more health care providers can educate themselves about this area of medicine, the better they will be able to provide the highest quality of care to their patients.

References

[1] NIH/NCCAM (National Institutes of Health/National Center for Complementary and Alternative Medicine). Meditation for health purposes. Available at: http://nccam.nih.gov/health/. Accessed February 2006.
[2] Han JS. Acupuncture and endorphins. Neurosci Lett 2004;361(1–3):258–61.
[3] Hui KK, Liu J, Makris N, et al. Acupuncture modulates the limbic system and subcortical gray structures of the human brain: evidence from fMRI studies in normal subjects. Hum Brain Mapp 2000;9(1):13–25.
[4] Berman BM, Ezzo J, Hadhazy V, et al. Is acupuncture effective in the treatment of fibromyalgia? J Fam Pract 1999;48(3):213–8.
[5] Guerra de Hoyas JA, Andres Martin Mdel C, Bassas y Baena de Leon E, et al. Randomised trial of long term effect of acupuncture for shoulder pain. Pain 2004;112(3):289–98.
[6] Trinh KV, Phillips SD, Ho E, et al. Acupuncture for the alleviation of lateral epicondyle pain: a systematic review. Rheumatol 2004;43(9):1085–90.
[7] Melchart D, Linde K, Fischer P, et al. Acupuncture for Idiopathic headaches. Cochrane Database Syst Rev 2001;1:CD001218.

[8] Melchart D, Streng A, Hoppe A, et al. Acupuncture for patients with tension-type headache: randomized control trial. BMJ 2005;331(7513):376–82.

[9] Linde K, Streng A, Jurgens S, et al. Acupuncture for patients with migraine: a randomized control trial. JAMA 2005;293(17):2118–25.

[10] Vickers A, Zollman C, McCarney R, et al. Acupuncture for chronic headache in primary care: large randomized trial. BMJ 2004;328:744–50.

[11] Backer M, Hammes M, Sander D, et al. Changes of cerebrovascular response to visual stimulation in migraineurs after repetitive session of somatosensory stimulation (acupuncture): a pilot study. Headache 2004;44(1):95–101.

[12] Irnich D, Behrens N, Gleditsh JM, et al. Immediate effects of dry needling and acupuncture at distant points in chronic neck pain: results of a randomized, double blinded, sham controlled crossover trial. Pain 2002;99(1–2):83–9.

[13] Witt C, Jena S, Brinkhaus B, et al. Acupuncture for patients with chronic neck pain. Pain 2006;125(1–2):98–106.

[14] Elden H, Ladfors L, Fagevik O, et al. Effects of acupuncture and stabilising exercises as adjunct to standard treatment in pregnant women with pelvic girdle pain: randomised single blind controlled trial. BMJ 2005;330(7494):761–6.

[15] Kvorning N, Holmberg C, Greenert L, et al. Acupuncture relieves pelvic and low back pain in late pregnancy. Acta Ostet Gynecol Scand 2004;83:246–50.

[16] Furlan AD, van Tulder MW, Cherkin DC, et al. Acupuncture and dry needling for low back pain. Cochrane Database Syst Rev 2005;1:CD001351.

[17] Manhelmer E, White A, Berman B, et al. Meta-analysis: acupuncture for low back pain. Ann Intern Med 2005;142:651–63.

[18] Brinkhaus B, Witt C, Jena S, et al. Acupuncture in patients with chronic low back pain. Arch Intern Med 2006;166:450–7.

[19] Molsberger A, Mau J, Pawelec D, et al. Does acupuncture improve the orthopedic management of chronic low back pain? A randomized, blinded, controlled trial with 3 months follow-up. Pain 2002;1999:579–87.

[20] Berman BM, Lao L, Langenberg P, et al. Effectiveness of acupuncture as adjunctive therapy in osteoarthritis of the knee. Ann Intern Med 2005;141(12):901–10.

[21] Linde K, Weidenhammer W, Streng A, et al. Acupuncture for osteoarthritic pain: an observational study in routine care. Rheumatol 2006;45:222–7.

[22] Vas J, Mendez C, Perea-Milla E, et al. Acupuncture as a complementary therapy to the pharmacological treatment of osteoarthritis of the knee: randomized controlled trial. BMJ 2004; 329:1216–21.

[23] Xia Q, Zhao KJ, Huang ZG, et al. Molecular genetic and chemical assessment of Rhizoma Curcumae in China. J Agric Food Chem 2005;53(15):6019–26.

[24] Arora RB, Kapoor V, Basu N, et al. Anti-inflammatory studies on Curcuma longa (turmeric). Indian J Med Res 1971;59:1289–95.

[25] Satoskar RR, Shah SJ, Shenoy SG. Evaluation of anti-inflammatory property of curcumin (diferoyl methane) in patients with postoperative inflammation. Int J Clin Pharmacol Ther Toxicol 1986;24(12):651–4.

[26] Ammon HPT, Wahl MA. Pharmacology of Curcuma longa. Planta Med 1991;57:1–7.

[27] Arora RB, Basu N, Kapoor V, et al. Anti-inflammatory studies on Curcuma longa (Turmeric). Indian J Med Res 1971;59(8):1289–95.

[28] Ramsewak RS, DeWitt DL, Nair MG. Cytotoxicity, antioxidant, and anti-inflammatory activities of Curcumins I–III from Curcuma longa. Phytomedicine 2000;7(4):303–8.

[29] Deodhar SD, Sethi R, Srimal RC. Preliminary study on antirheumatic activity of curcumin (diferoyl methane). Indian J Med Res 1980;71:632–4.

[30] Altman RD, Marcussen KC. Effects of a ginger extract on knee pain in patients with osteoarthritis. Arthritis Rheum 2001;44(11):2531–8.

[31] Bliddal H, Rosetzky A, Schlichting P, et al. A randomized, placebo-controlled, cross-over study of ginger extracts and ibuprofen in osteoarthritis. Osteoarthritis Cartilage 2000;8:9–12.

[32] Chrubasik S. Pain therapy using herbal medicines. Gynakologe 2000;33(1):59–64.

[33] Schmid B, Ludtke R, Selbmann HK, et al. Efficacy and tolerability of a standardized willow bark extract in patients with osteoarthritis: randomized placebo-controlled, double blind clinical trial. Phytotherapy Research 2001;15(4):344–50.

[34] Schnitzer TJ, Morton C, Coker S, et al. Effectiveness of reduced applications of topical capsaicin (0.025-percent) in osteoarthritis. Arthritis and Rheumatism 1992;35(9):S132.

[35] McCarthy GM, McCarty DL. Effect of topical capsaicin in the therapy of painful osteoarthritis of the hands. J Rheumatol 1992;19:604–7.

[36] Altman RD, Aven A, Holmburg CE, et al. Capsaicin cream 0.025% as monotherapy for osteoarthritis: a double-blind study. Semin Arthritis Rheum 1994;23(Suppl):25–33.

[37] Ammon HP, Safayhi H, Mack T, et al. Mechanism of antiinflammatory actions of curcumine and boswellic acids. J Ethnopharmacol 1993;38:113–9.

[38] Kulkarni RRPP, Jog VP, Gandage SG, et al. Treatment of osteoarthritis with herbomineral formulation: a double-blind, placebo-controlled, cross-over study. J Ethnopharmacol 1991; 33:91–5.

[39] Chopra A, Lavin P, Patwardhan B, et al. Randomized double blind trial of an ayurvedic plant derived formulation for treatment of rheumatoid arthritis. J Rheumatol 2000;27: 1365–72.

[40] Basch E, Foppa I, Liebowitz R, et al. Lavender (Lavandula angustifolia Miller). J Herb Pharmacother 2004;4(2):63–78.

[41] Lis-Balchin M, Hart S. Studies on the mode of action of the essential oil of Lavender (Lavendula angustifolia p. Miller). Phytother Res 1999;13(6):540–2.

[42] Gedney JJ, Glover TL, Fillingim RB. Sensory and affective pain discrimination after inhalation of essential oils. Psychosom Med 2004;66(4):599–606.

[43] Sumner H, Salan U, Knight D, et al. Inhibition of 5-lipoxygenase and cyclo-oxygenase in leukocytes by feverfew. Involvement of sesquiterpene lactones and other components. Biochem Pharmacol 1992;43(11):2313–20.

[44] Volger BK, Pittler MH, Ernst E. Feverfew as a preventive treatment for migraine: a systemic review. Cephalagia 1998;18:704–8.

Manual Therapy References

[45] Eisenberg DM, Davis RB, Ettner SL, et al. Trends in alternative medicine use in the United States, 1990–1997: results of a follow-up national survey. JAMA 1998;280(18): 1569–75.

[46] Astin JA. Why patients use alternative medicine: results of a national study. JAMA 1998; 279(19):1548–53.

[47] Panjabi MM. A hypothesis of chronic back pain: ligament subfailure injuries lead to muscle control dysfunction. Eur Spine J 2006;15(5):668–76.

[48] Melzack R. From the gate to the neuromatrix. Pain 1999;(Suppl 6):S121–6.

[49] Villanueva L, Le Bars D. Activation of bulbo-spinal controls by peripheral nociceptive inputs: diffuse noxious inhibitory controls. Biol Res 1995;28(1):113–25.

[50] Meeker WC, Haldeman S. Chiropractic: a profession at the crossroads of mainstream and alternative medicine. Ann Intern Med 2002;136(3):216–27.

[51] Assendelft WJ, Morton SC, Yu EI, et al. Spinal manipulative therapy for low back pain. Cochrane Database Syst Rev 2004;1:CD000447.

[52] Cherkin DC, Deyo RA, Battie M, et al. A comparison of physical therapy, chiropractic manipulation, and provision of an educational booklet for the treatment of patients with low back pain. N Engl J Med 1998;339(15):1021–9.

[53] Waddell G, Newton M, Henderson I, et al. Fear-Avoidance Beliefs Questionnaire (FABQ) and the role of fear-avoidance beliefs in chronic low back pain and disability. Pain 1993; 52(2):157–68.

[54] Childs JD, Fritz JM, Flynn TW, et al. A clinical prediction rule to identify patients with low back pain most likely to benefit from spinal manipulation: a validation study. Ann Intern Med 2004;141(12):920–8.

[55] Andersson GB, Lucente T, Davis AM, et al. A comparison of osteopathic spinal manipulation with standard care for patients with low back pain. N Engl J Med 1999;341(19):1426–31.

[56] Williams NH, Wilkinson C, Russell I, et al. Randomized osteopathic manipulation study (ROMANS): pragmatic trial for spinal pain in primary care. Fam Pract 2003;20(6):662–9.

[57] Klougart N, Leboeuf-Yde C, Rasmussen LR. Safety in chiropractic practice. Part II: Treatment to the upper neck and the rate of cerebrovascular incidents. J Manipulative Physiol Ther 1996;19(9):563–9.

[58] Koes BW, Assendelft WJ, van der Heijden GJ, et al. Spinal manipulation for low back pain. An updated systematic review of randomized clinical trials. Spine 1996;21(24):2860–71 [discussion 2872–3].

[59] Kapral MK, Bondy SJ. Cervical manipulation and risk of stroke. CMAJ 2001;165(7):907–8.

[60] Lund I, Ge Y, Yu LC, et al. Repeated massage-like stimulation induces long-term effects on nociception: contribution of oxytocinergic mechanisms. Eur J Neurosci 2002;16(2):330–8.

[61] Cherkin DC, Sherman KJ, Deyo RA, et al. A review of the evidence for the effectiveness, safety, and cost of acupuncture, massage therapy, and spinal manipulation for back pain. Ann Intern Med 2003;138(11):898–906.

[62] Cherkin DC, Eisenberg D, Sherman KJ, et al. Randomized trial comparing traditional Chinese medical acupuncture, therapeutic massage, and self-care education for chronic low back pain. Arch Intern Med 2001;161(8):1081–8.

[63] Hernandez-Reif M, Field T, Krasnegor J, et al. Lower back pain is reduced and range of motion increased after massage therapy. Int J Neurosci 2001;106(3–4):131–45.

[64] Preyde M. Effectiveness of massage therapy for subacute low-back pain: a randomized controlled trial. CMAJ 2000;162(13):1815–20.

[65] Irnich D, Behrens N, Molzen H, et al. Randomised trial of acupuncture compared with conventional massage and "sham" laser acupuncture for treatment of chronic neck pain. BMJ 2001;322(7302):1574–8.

[66] Field T, Diego M, Cullen C, et al. Fibromyalgia pain and substance P decrease and sleep improves after massage therapy. J Clin Rheumatol 2002;8(2):72–6.

[67] Vuori IM. Dose-response of physical activity and low back pain, osteoarthritis, and osteoporosis. Med Sci Sports Exerc 2001;33(6 Suppl):S551–86.

[68] Hoffman MD, Shepanski MA, Mackenzie SP, et al. Experimentally induced pain perception is acutely reduced by aerobic exercise in people with chronic low back pain. J Rehabil Res Dev 2005;42(2):183–90.

[69] Koltyn KF. Analgesia following exercise: a review. Sports Med 2000;29(2):85–98.

[70] Adreani CM, Hill JM, Kaufman MP. Responses of group III and IV muscle afferents to dynamic exercise. J Appl Physiol 1997;82(6):1811–7.

[71] Williams KA, Petronis J, Smith D, et al. Effect of Iyengar yoga therapy for chronic low back pain. Pain 2005;115(1–2):107–17.

[72] Sherman KJ, Cherkin DC, Erro J, et al. Comparing yoga, exercise, and a self-care book for chronic low back pain: a randomized, controlled trial. Ann Intern Med 2005;143(12):849–56.

[73] Lan C, Chen SY, Lai JS. Relative exercise intensity of Tai Chi Chuan is similar in different ages and gender. Am J Chin Med 2004;32(1):151–60.

[74] Audette JF, Jin YS, Newcomer R, et al. Tai Chi versus brisk walking in elderly women. Age Ageing 2006;35(4):388–93.

[75] Hartman CA, Manos TM, Winter C, et al. Effects of T'ai Chi training on function and quality of life indicators in older adults with osteoarthritis. J Am Geriatr Soc 2000;48:1553–9.

[76] Song R, Lee EO, Lam P, et al. Effects of tai chi exercise on pain, balance, muscle strength, and perceived difficulties in physical functioning in older women with osteoarthritis: a randomized clinical trial. J Rheumatol 2003;30(9):2039–44.

[77] Wenk-Sormaz H. Meditation can reduce habitual responding. Adv Mind Body Med 2005; 21:33–49.

[78] Benson H. Timeless Healing: The Power and Biology of Belief. New York: Scribner; 1996.

[79] Mamtani R, Cimino A. A primer of complementary and alternative medicine and its relevance in the treatment of mental health problems. Psychiatr Q 2002;73:367–81.

[80] Schaffer SD, Yucha CB. Relaxation and pain management: the relaxation response can play a role in managing chronic and acute pain. Am J Nurs 2004;104:75–82.

[81] Newberg AB, Iversen J. The neural basis of the complex mental task of meditation: neurotransmitter and neurochemical considerations. Med Hypotheses 2003;61:282–91.

[82] Travis F. Autonomic and EEG patterns distinguish transcending from other experiences during transcendental meditation practice. Int J Psychophysiol 2001;42:1–9.

[83] Perez-de-Albenez A, Holmes J. Meditation: concepts, effects, and uses in therapy. Int J Psychother 2000;5:49–58.

[84] Walsh R, Shapiro SL. The meeting of meditative disciplines and western psychology: a mutually enriching dialogue. Am Psychol 2006;61:227–39.

[85] Jevning R, Wallace RK, Biedebach M. The physiology of meditation: a review: a wakeful hypometabolic integrated response. Neurosci Biobehav Rev 1992;16:415–24.

[86] Jacobs GD. Clinical applications of the relaxation response and mind-body interventions. J Altern Complement Med 2001;7(S1):S93–101.

[87] Peng CK, Mietus JE, Liu Y, et al. Exaggerated heart rate oscillations during two meditation techniques. Int J Cardiol 1999;70:101–7.

[88] Baer RA. Mindfulness training as a clinical intervention: a conceptual and empirical review. Clin Psychol Sci Pract 2003;10:125–43.

[89] Caspi O, Burleson KO. Methodological challenges in meditation research. Adv Mind Body Med 2005;21:4–11.

[90] Rainville P, Duncan GH, Price DD, et al. Pain affect encoded in human anterior cingulate but not somatosensory cortex. Science 1997;277:968–71.

[91] Rainville P, Bao QVH, Chretien P. Pain-related emotions modulate experimental pain perception and autonomic responses. Pain 2005;118(3):306–18.

[92] Rainville P, Carrier B, Hofbauer RK, et al. Dissociation of sensory and affective dimensions of pain using hypnotic modulation. Pain 1999;82:159–71.

[93] Kiernan BD, Dane JR, Philips LH, et al. Hypnotic analgesia reduces R-III nociceptive reflex: further evidence concerning the multifactorial nature of hypnotic analgesia. Pain 1995;60: 39–47.

[94] Lang EV, Benotsch EG, Fick LJ, et al. Adjunctive non-pharmacologic analgesia for invasive medical procedures: a randomized trial. Lancet 2000;355:1486–90.

[95] Jensen M, Patterson DR. Hypnotic treatment of chronic pain. J Behav Med 2006;29(1): 95–124.

[96] Haanen HC, Hoenderdos HT, van Romunde LK, et al. Controlled trial of hypnotherapy in the treatment of refractory fibromyalgia. J Rheumatol 1991;18(1):72–5.

[97] Gay MC, Philippot P, Luminet O. Differential effectiveness of psychological interventions for reducing osteoarthritis pain: a comparison of Erikson [correction of Erickson] hypnosis and Jacobson relaxation. Eur J Pain 2002;6(1):1–16.

[98] Friedman H, Taub HA. Brief psychological training procedures in migraine treatment. Am J Clin Hypn 1984;26(3):187–200.

ELSEVIER
SAUNDERS

Med Clin N Am 91 (2007) 169–176

THE MEDICAL
CLINICS
OF NORTH AMERICA

Index

Note: Page numbers of article titles are in **boldface** type.

Quantitative sudomotor axon reflex test, 26

Quebec Task Force, 38–40

Qugong breathing exercises, 158–159

R

Range of motion
evaluation of, 64–65
stretching of, 71

Recreation therapy, 70–71

Rehabilitation, physiatric model of.
See Physiatric model of care.

Relaxation
in cognitive-behavioral therapy, 48–49
in meditation, 159–160

RICE (rest, ice, compression, and
elevation), 59

Rofecoxib, 101–102, 107, 109–110

Rostral medial medulla, in pain
transmission, 7–8

S

Salicylates, 103–105

Saskatchewan Government Insurance data,
40–41

Selective serotonin reuptake inhibitors, 87,
114

Self-efficacy beliefs, in behavioral
therapy, 50

Sensitization, 6–8
central, 3
of nociceptors, 2

Sensory nerve action potential, 25

Sensory testing, quantitative, 25–26

Serotonin norepinephrine dual-reuptake
inhibitors, 87, 114

Shoulder pain, acupuncture for, 149–150

Single-leg stance test, for core strength, 66

Skin biopsy, in neuropathic pain, 27

Sleep disorders, in fibromyalgia, 86

Slump test, in back pain, 82

Sodium channels, tricyclic antidepressant
interaction with, 129–130

Spinal cord, pain signal transmission in, 2–4

Spinal manipulative therapy, 153–156

Spinal sensitization, 6–8

Spray and stretch technique, for myofascial
pain syndrome, 85

Stability, evaluation of, 66–67

Stabilization exercise, for back pain, 80–81

Stagnation, as pathogenic factor, 148

Stomach, damage of, due to NSAIDs,
100–101

Strength, evaluation of, 65–66

Stress reduction, behavioral therapy for,
45–55

Stretching exercises, 71, 85

Stroke, in manipulative therapies, 155–156

Substance P, in pain transmission, 3

Sulindac, 108

T

Tai chi, 73, 158–159

Taxonomy, of pain, **13–20**

Tender points, in fibromyalgia, 86

TENS (transcutaneous electrical
stimulation), 73–75
for myofascial pain syndrome, 85
for osteoarthritis, 80

Thalidomide, 119

Thermoregulatory sweat test, 26

Thrombosis disorders, due to NSAIDs,
101–102

Tiagabine, 115

Tizanidine, 116

Tolmetin, 108

Topical analgesics, 117, **125–139**
alpha-adrenoreceptor antagonists, 132
antidepressants, 129–131
anti-inflammatory agents, 126–127
cannabinoids, 132
capsaicin, 117, 128–129
glutamate receptor antagonists,
131–132
local anesthetics, 127–128
opioids, 132–133

Topiramate, 115

Traditional Chinese Medicine
acupuncture in, 142–152
herbal formulas in, 152–153

Transcutaneous electrical stimulation,
73–75

Transcutaneous (*continued*)
  for myofascial pain syndrome, 85
  for osteoarthritis, 80

Transduction, in pain neural processing, 2

Transmission, in pain neural processing, 2–3

Trendelenberg's sign, 66, 68

Tricyclic antidepressants, 113–114, 129–131

Trigeminal neuralgia, 24

Trigger points, in myofascial pain
  syndrome, 82–85

Tumor necrosis factor-alpha inhibitors, 119

U

Ulcers, due to NSAIDs, 100–101

Ultrasound therapy, 76–77

Upper-crossed syndrome, 65

V

Valdecoxib, 101–102, 107, 109–110

Venlafaxine, 87, 114

Vertebral artery dissection, in manipulative
  therapies, 155–156

W

Waddell symptoms and signs of illness
  behavior, 62–63

Whiplash injuries, task force on, 38–40

Whirlpool therapy, 76

Wind, as pathogenic factor, 145–146

Wind-Cold syndrome, 145–146

Wind-Damp syndrome, 146

Wind-Heat syndrome, 145–146

Workers compensation, 33

Y

Yin and yang, in acupuncture, 144–148

Yoga, 158

Z

Zang organs, in acupuncture, 144–145

Zolendronic acid, 118

Zonisamide, 115

Moving?

Make sure your subscription moves with you!

To notify us of your new address, find your **Clinics Account Number** (located on your mailing label above your name), and contact customer service at:

E-mail: elspcs@elsevier.com

800-654-2452 (subscribers in the U.S. & Canada)
407-345-4000 (subscribers outside of the U.S. & Canada)

Fax number: 407-363-9661

Elsevier Periodicals Customer Service
6277 Sea Harbor Drive
Orlando, FL 32887-4800

*To ensure uninterrupted delivery of your subscription, please notify us at least 4 weeks in advance of move.